THE AVOCADO SHOW

PRESENTS THE AVOCADO BOOK

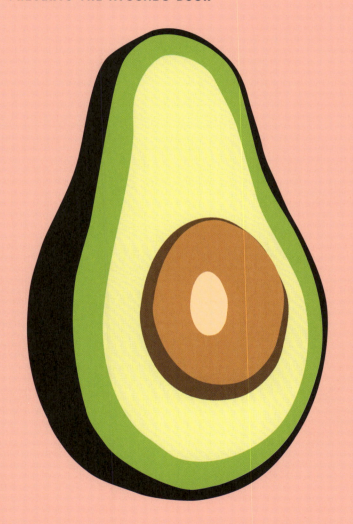

RECIPES FOR THE WORLD'S MOST INSTAGRAMMABLE FRUIT
PRETTY HEALTHY FOOD WITH FOODDECO

PAVILION

LET THE SHOW BEGIN

The Avocado Show is one of the most exciting food start-ups in the world. What began as a single restaurant in Amsterdam with only 45 seats, grew into the world's first avocado franchise concept within a year, with hundreds of thousands of online and offline fans. Of course, we knew what we were doing, but this was something nobody really expected.

So who are "we" then? Apologies. HI THERE! We're Ron Simpson and Julien Zaal, two friends from Amsterdam who played records together, made some music, threw lots of parties, and tried to make life a little more fun for ourselves and those around us.

We didn't know much about restaurants. Yet when it came to awesome events, great brands and viral marketing, we knew plenty. When we came up with the idea to open a mono restaurant that would focus on beautiful avocado dishes – because it's our favourite superfruit – everyone thought we were mad. But we had no doubts. The avocado is not only really delicious, it is also versatile and lends itself to the most beautiful creations. We decided to take the risk and five days later we had the keys to our new restaurant (read: adventure) in our hands.

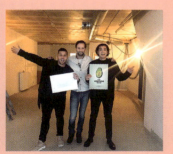

The photo that started all the madness.

We had no idea what was in store for us. If you would have told us that fans would camp out and sleep on our doorstep, that there would be queues going round the corner every day, and that millions of people would be looking at our photos and videos, we would have never believed you. But it couldn't be more true!

Before sending out an official press release, we first wanted to break the good news to our friends and family through Facebook and Instagram. Using a mobile phone, we took a quick snapshot inside our empty building, and as soon as we put it online, the madness began. Our idea went viral like a celebrity sex tape! While we did expect to get love and attention from the people around us, we were taken by surprise when suddenly our news was published in 60 different countries and

"OUR IDEA WENT VIRAL LIKE A CELEBRITY SEX TAPE!"

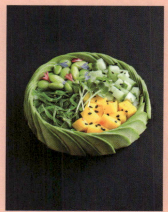

The most beautiful poke bowl in the world. Even if we say so ourselves.

20 different languages, our videos were watched hundreds of millions of times, and we received all kinds of interview requests from every corner of the world!

We appeared in Japanese game shows, the Chinese news, the front page in Australia, the biggest newspapers in New York, documentaries in Germany and so much more. Every day we were tagged just about everywhere, and suddenly the phone rang with a number from Dubai: would we be interested in opening a branch on the Palm Islands? Man, it just kept getting crazier. The first franchise request was made, and hundreds would follow in the first few weeks.

But what did they actually want to franchise? We didn't have anything yet! Except for a good idea, that is. The time was ripe for us to develop our menu with the help of our good friend and superstar chef Jaimie van Heije. We also got tons of inspiration online from Colette Dike of Fooddeco, who helped us realise our dreams from the start. We knew that each dish had to be 50 per cent about the avocado and 50 per cent about the show. It had to be delicious, of course, but also stunning to look at. Yummy first, beautiful second, and served in a restaurant with plenty of style, enabling you to be the photographer. The search for Pretty Healthy Food had started!

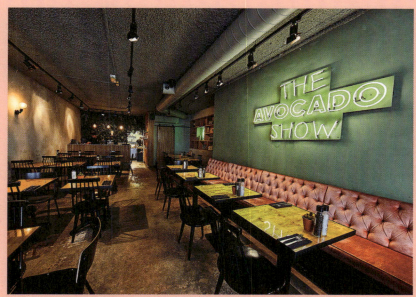

Good vibes only! The now world-famous pink sofa, plant walls and neon.

How do we avocado it? That was the question we asked ourselves every day. Take your favourite dish, tack on that question, and you'll know how we did it. Pizza. How do we avocado it? Hamburgers. How do we avocado it? Pancakes. How do we avocado it? All the classics were considered, and we tried just about anything imaginable. Not everything was equally good, but some dishes were instant classics. There was a perfect union between avocado and poached eggs, the salads became even greener, the poke bowls looked like masterpieces, and you couldn't order toasts like ours anywhere else in the world. Who would've thought the avocado could be so versatile? It was almost impossible to choose which dishes would make it to the menu – we wanted them all!

There was one thing we were sure of: if we couldn't get good avocados every day, this party wasn't going to happen. We all had the same conditions and wishes: ripe, sustainable and socially sound avocados. And they can only be found at one place: Nature's Pride.

We came into contact with Nature's Pride when a marketeer posted our restaurant on their Facebook page and they got a hundred times more likes than normal. After they had tried to get in touch with us a few times, we decided to stop by and have a look. WHAT. A. COMPANY. WOW! How they handled the fruit was already remarkable, but how they dealt with people was truly impressive. From order picker to avocado grower and Mother Earth, everyone was taken into account and cared for. A philosophy which we immediately adhered to and felt comfortable with.

Besides all the love, we also got messages and questions about the sustainability of avocados. How much water does it take to grow them? What is the impact of transport? And how about all the news items from Mexico? We had no idea, but we wanted to know everything ourselves as well, of course. After conducting a lot of online research, but not being satisfied with the answers, we decided to go on a quest for the truth.

We follow every step of our avocados, from the tree to your plate!

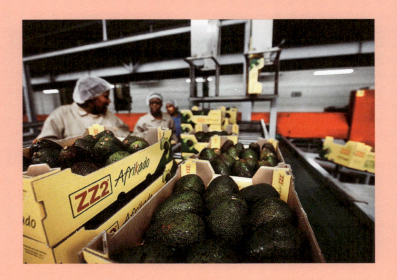

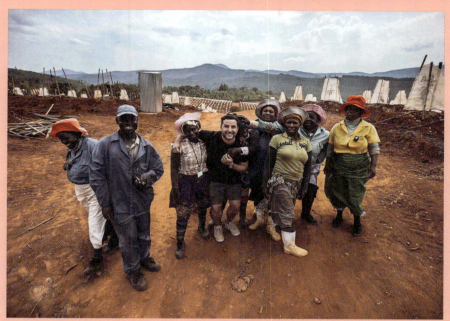
Work hard, play hard. Everyone walks around with a smile. We do too.

"WE DECIDED TO GO ON A QUEST FOR THE TRUTH OURSELVES"

We visited the farmers and countries that supply Nature's Pride with the avocados we sell in our restaurant. Along the way, we learned everything about growing avocados: we researched water use in Chile, social developments in Peru, working conditions in South Africa and the rumours in Mexico.

We learned that in the right areas, avocados could grow using rainwater and that the avocado allows certain economies to prosper fully: schools and hospitals are being built; employees are queueing every year for well-paid jobs; and some farmers and communities help up to 80,000 people in their neighbourhood.

With pride and joy, we witnessed how sustainability, water use and socially responsible entrepreneurship were of utmost importance for every grower we visited. We were allowed to see everything, ask everything and know everything; everyone was willing to talk to us about better solutions and ideas. Of course, there's still plenty of room for improvement in the entire industry and we're all working hard on that, but our supplier has taken care of it down to the smallest detail, just as we would aim to do ourselves. And that's something we're proud of.

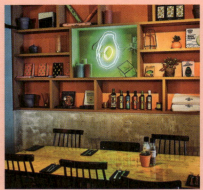

Avocado cosmetics, umbrellas, books, kitchen tools, and much more at our wannahave Avo Wall.

Back in the Netherlands, we found ourselves in another crazy situation. Because of all the media attention, people assumed we were already open! Every day, hundreds of people travelled from all over the world to knock on our closed doors, eager to have a bite. But there wasn't even a single chair inside. What could we do about that? We decided to set up everything ourselves and open our doors as soon as possible. We chose the famous pink sofa, the green plant walls, the tables and chairs, and every other detail in the establishment ourselves. We opened the doors to our first restaurant on March 17th, 2017. Was everything perfect? Absolutely not. But it was great fun!

We thought it would be fun to raffle the first spots to our fans, but suddenly there were 22,000 registrations and only 45 available seats. It took us about a week to reply to everyone, but the first day was unforgettable and the queue that appeared has been returning ever since.

˙22,000 REGISTRATIONS AND ONLY 45 SEATS˙

Everyone enjoys the food, the drinks, the good vibes, and the crazy playlists we put together ourselves. Our fantastic, international staff know how to combine service with character, and they turn every day into a party. It's still so awesome to see everyone who comes in taking pictures of the place or of the beautiful dishes. It just makes us so happy.

The story keeps getting better, the days more fun and the ideas crazier. Next to the restaurant, we also created and curated some merchandise, just for fun: We sell The Avocado Show T-shirts and hoodies, as well as avocado Christmas balls, bathrobes, cookbooks, cooking oil, pins, and phone cases. And that's how the world's first avocado pop-up store came about!

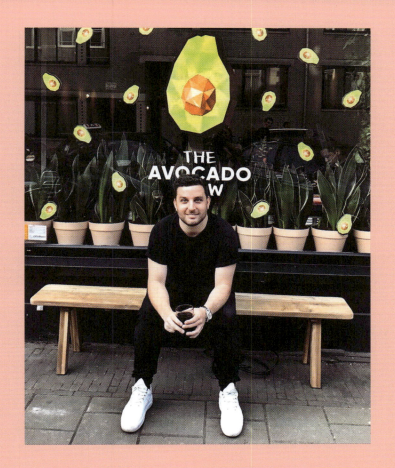

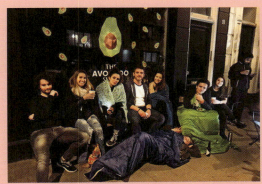

These avocado fans slept in front of the door the night before the opening. Incredible!

We've put together a collection of the coolest avocado stuff on the planet, which you can find at each location and through our online shop, from where we send products to just about every country in the world. It doesn't matter who or where you are; the love for avocados is truly universal. We hope a package will go to Mars one day.

In order to make our dreams come true and open The Avocado Show in every cool city in the world, we needed help. Not just an investment to develop and finance everything, but also a lot of knowledge, experience and support. And who knows more about our favourite green fruit in the world than the Bill Gates of avocados: Shawn Harris? Nobody. Nobody? Nope, nobody.

During a fantastic test dinner with our new dishes, we shared our vision, all our crazy ideas, possibilities and opportunities with this lady. No holding back, all cards on the table. A bit daring, but hey, we were so enthusiastic that we couldn't contain ourselves. The following day we got a really simple, but very clear email: LET'S DO IT.

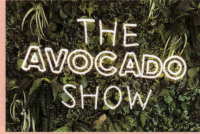

Our love for green is hard to miss!

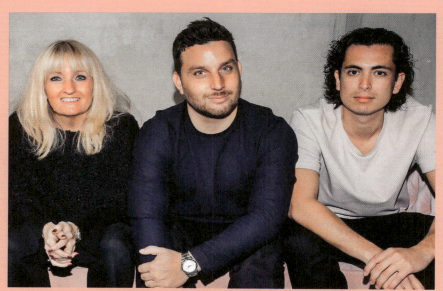

Working together with the lady who made the avocado great is always a good idea.

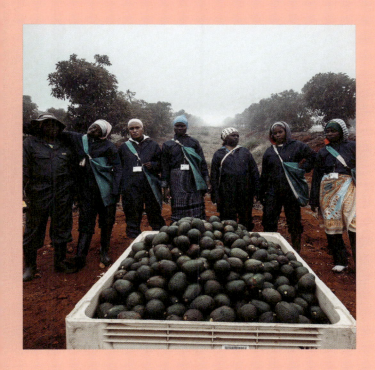

The collaboration was born – we had found the best partner one could wish for and could go on thinking about our future. And the future is definitely green. No question about that. We believe The Avocado Show is an international brand which deserves a place in every cool city in the world. Sometimes in the form of a complete restaurant where lucky avocado fans can eat just about any avocado dish they can imagine, and sometimes in the form of a Boutique where we can promise every district "Pretty Healthy Food for the Neighbourhood". Delicious, beautiful and healthy food that's easily available at any time of the day.

We believe that, together with our suppliers, friends and fans, we can help improve sustainability, promote responsible farming, and reduce the environmental impact of producing avocados all over the world – by setting high standards for our own suppliers, as well as by setting up our own projects to promote sustainability and reduce waste.

Our aim is to do great things, meet nice people and make the world a better place, whilst getting the most out of avocados – and all with a smile.

We are incredibly grateful for all your time, interest, support and love. Why don't you stop by for a bite soon? That would be awesome!

The Avocado Show Team

"THE FUTURE IS DEFINITELY GREEN"

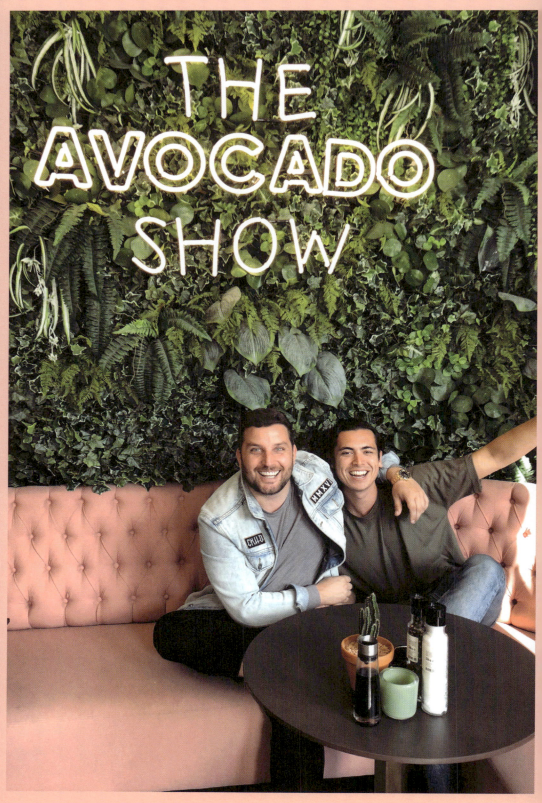

PRETTY HEALTHY FOOD

"A DISH
SHOULD BE
FULL OF
FLAVOUR
AND ALSO
BEAUTIFULLY
PRESENTED"

The works of art we serve at The Avocado Show are so much more than just delicious avocado dishes served on beautiful plates. Every day we lavish them with endless amounts of love, time and attention, and are constantly developing new ideas.

Before we put one of our creations on the menu, it has to meet all of the requirements of our **Pretty Healthy Food** concept.

Pretty Healthy Food means that a dish should be full of flavour and also beautifully presented, that every dish should be nutritious, and that the experience should make you happy. This goes for the food served in the restaurant as well as for all of the tasty takeaway items eaten at home.

We consider every element – the tableware, the packaging, the cutlery, the forms, the colours, the patterns, the contrast, the experience, and so much more – to turn every dish into a real event.

Our ideas come from far and wide, and we're surrounded by a fantastic team that is constantly coming up with innovative concepts. Professional chefs, enthusiastic fans, dedicated staff, and our own obsession with avocados make sure there's always a new challenge waiting to be seized.

One of our favourite food creators is Colette Dike of Fooddeco. Her presentation style, choice of colours, originality and creativity are second to none, as also evidenced by her huge host of online fans.

We had the honour of working along with the Fooddeco team to put together a selection of beautiful and tasty dishes for this gorgeous book, many of them our own favourites. From classics to fancy fast food, and from sweet to savoury: it's all here.

We've paid special attention to all the various lifestyle choices, so there are options for vegans, flexitarians, vegetarians, pescatarians, and more! We love you all.

We hope you enjoy the recipes, take pleasure in preparing them and share what you make with your friends.

We look forward to seeing you soon in one of our locations!

Ron & Julien

WE ARE NATURE'S PRIDE

Nature's Pride supplies over 250 unique fruits and vegetables from 70 countries. From ready-to-eat and exotic fruit and vegetables to the delicious berries and off season products. Together with our partners, we make a difference every day. The quality of our products is a result of many factors: from the passion of the grower, our dedicated employees and our unique expertise in the ripening of fruit to an appealing presentation on our customers' shelves. This is how we make sure we supply optimum quality fruit and vegetables that people can enjoy every day.

FOUNDED BY SHAWN HARRIS IN 2001

--FIRST--

MANGO & AVOCADO RIPENERS IN EUROPE

WOW!

In Mexico, 10 kilos of avocado get eaten per person per year

WORLD RECORD

THE WORLD RECORD FOR THE LARGEST AVOCADO IS 5 POUNDS 3.6 OUNCES.

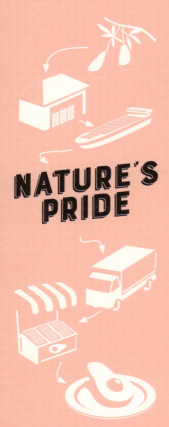

NATURE'S PRIDE

WHAT MAKES THEM TICK?

Delivering the most unique and tasty fruits & vegetables to their customers and making the world more sustainable and healthy.

THE EXOTIC FRUIT - AND - VEGETABLE EXPERT - IN - EUROPE

THE WORD "GUACAMOLE" IS FROM THE AZTEC WORD "ĀHUACAMOLLI", WHICH LITERALLY MEANS "AVOCADO SAUCE"

AMAZING

AMAZING

AMAZING

AMAZING

Avocados are a symbol of love and fertility in Aztec culture

Next to avocados and mangos, the people at NP have big love for

BERRIES!

250 PRODUCTS

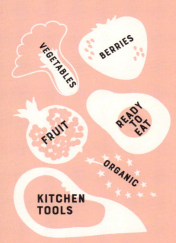

VEGETABLES

BERRIES

FRUIT

READY TO EAT

ORGANIC

KITCHEN TOOLS

THE SECRET OF READY TO EAT

How do they manage to give their avocados such a creamy and nutty taste? Growers postpone the harvest of avocados until the fruits have a perfect oil content. The avocados are picked on average two weeks later than other avocados you'll find in store.

UNIQUE

In partnership with the growers, Nature's Pride goes far beyond the minimum social requirements and enables workers and communities to prosper.

Nature's Pride's Sustainable Business team – as well as its commercial staff – know the growers well. Focussed on sustainability, they build partnerships with full commitment and dedication. They take health seriously at NP, not only by eating **nutritious avocados,** but also by building their own **outdoor fitness area** to improve the health and well-being of all employees.

Nature's Pride contributes to a better world with its passion and experience. Putting people at the heart of its operations and working on the development of communities and the protection of the environment.

The Nature's Pride Foundation finances local projects in communities where they grow the fruit and vegetables. The aim is to stimulate economic growth of small farmers, pack-house employees and their families.

RIPE ~ IN ~ STORE

READY TO ENJOY AT HOME RIGHT AWAY

PASSION INNOVATIVE COMMITTED CREATIVE HEALTHY SUSTAINABLE PIONEER HONEST DEDICATED TOGETHER OPEN

400 GROWERS ACROSS 70 COUNTRIES

SUPPLY OUR PRODUCTS TO

28 COUNTRIES

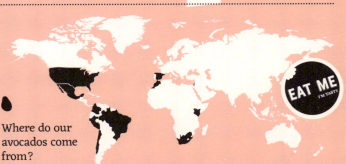

EAT ME
I'M TASTY

Where do our avocados come from?

FOODDECO & COLETTE

"OVER 40 DELICIOUS AND BEAUTIFUL DISHES FOR EVERY MOMENT OF THE DAY"

I never get tired of avocados. My love for avocados is actually a pregnancy craving that got out of hand. When I was pregnant with my first child, I made more and more things with avocado, and was always experimenting. I took it as a challenge to present avocados in ways that were new, original and, above all, easy. This started with the avocado ribbons and the avocado burger bun, followed by sushicado, the avocado garden, and others. The photos of these creations became instant internet sensations, and a number of them are now served at The Avocado Show and other restaurants. So special!

Because the avocado is so incredibly versatile, I've got ideas to spare. I hope these recipes will inspire you to work with this remarkable fruit. For you and your sweetheart, for your children, for your family and friends, for anyone you choose: avocado fits well into any part of any meal, no matter what time of day. I even spread avocado on my bread instead of butter. Delicious!

I want to encourage people to make food that is tasty and healthy, and also food that looks beautiful without too much effort. That's why this book contains recipes and tips and tricks for making your homemade dishes that little bit more exciting and attractive. And seriously: you can do it!

I also don't want to burden you with a long list of ingredients that your local supermarket might not carry. Things shouldn't be too complicated. Another important consideration is 'no waste': use everything to the greatest extent possible. For example, I also make use of broccoli stems, as you can see on page 66. And it doesn't end there: don't just use the gherkins or pickled onions from the jar – make sure you save the liquid, too. It's a shame to throw it away because you can put this to good use for flavouring another dish.

This book contains over 40 delicious and beautiful dishes for every moment of the day, with lots of (styling) tips and how-to's. Together with The Avocado Show, we've compiled our avocado creations, ideas, and experiences – a process that has resulted in this wonderful pink book.

So enjoy this amazing fruit! There's a reason it's known as 'green gold'.

Love,
xoxo

Colette
a.k.a Fooddeco

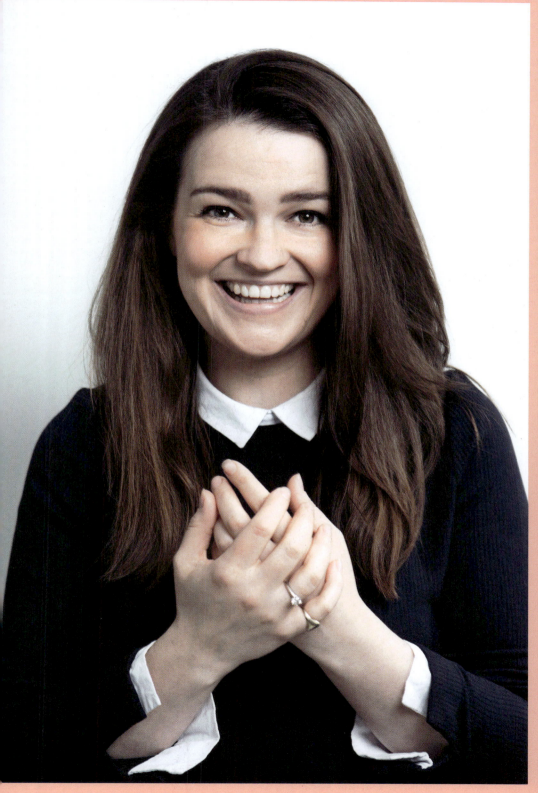

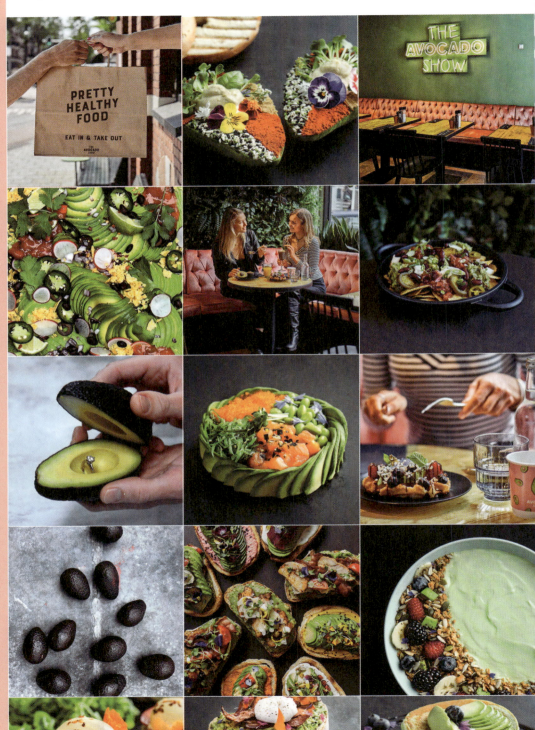

#AVOCADO

A quick search shows nearly 10 million uses of #avocado worldwide, making it one of the most popular food items on Instagram. #avocadotoast is also high on the list with nearly one million hashtags. That's one reason this book contains no less than six variations on the classic 'avocado on toast'. The beloved avocado now even has its own emoticon.

People love the avocado for its flavour and nutrients, but also because it's incredibly photogenic. It makes any food photo more appealing. In addition, it lends itself as a key ingredient to all kinds of dishes, from original breakfasts to desserts. And there's something for everyone. Vegetarians, vegans and diehard carnivores will be surprised and delighted.

The popularity of the avocado on Instagram goes beyond just photos. For example, the avocado proposal of Fooddeco is one of my most popular posts, and even went viral internationally. Since then, #avocadoproposal has featured in many marriage proposals around the world.

From mashed avocados on toast to avocado gardens and avocado roses: you'll see the avocado presented in a multitude of forms in this book. Have you ever tried making an avocado rose? It's easier than you think – have a look on page 136 for a 'how-to'.

Show the world what you've got and don't forget to tag us: @theavocadoshow and @fooddeco or #theavocadoshow and #fooddecoavocado. You'll find lots of inspiration and brilliant recipes on our timelines, so why don't you hit that follow button?

THE MENU

The avocado's versatility means it's possible to dream up something delicious for every moment of the day. We've divided all of the goodness into seven categories.

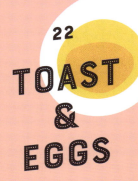

22
TOAST & EGGS

Try to name a more iconic duo. We'll wait…

48
BOWLS & SALADS

Avocado gives every salad more flair. Its velvety richness turns even the simplest salad into one that is sumptuous and substantial, as well as being nourishing. Avocados also make the perfect 'bowl', like the poke bowls on page 50.

36
AVOCADO GARDENS

If you're always looking for new ways to present a dish that is both attractive and easy to achieve, these avocado gardens are an excellent example. Simplicity itself – you serve avocado halves (with the pit and peel removed), using the hollow that held the pit to hold a tasty sauce or your choice of hummus, and decorate the top of the avocado half. An instant eye-catcher without too much effort.

64
FANCY FAST FOOD

Following the success of the avocado burger and the delicious – and healthier – avocado chips (fries), other versions of familiar fast food dishes based on avocado were bound to emerge. The deliciously rich and creamy flavour of avocado makes it an excellent substitute for 'greasy' snacks. We just can't get enough of the avo nuggets (see page 68), the avocado frites sauce (see page 70), and the avo satay skewers (see page 76).

84
CLASSICS

You're probably familiar with classic dishes – especially French ones – including steak tartare and hollandaise sauce (try to make this in 60 seconds flat – check it out on page 88). There are also many wonderful classic Italian dishes, including gnocchi (see page 98). Good news for all avocado aficionados out there: avocados can be combined very well with some of these dishes to create classics with a twist.

102
SNACK-
BAR

The most famous dip ever could well be guacamole. The basis for guacamole is mashed avocado flavoured with various ingredients, from chilli flakes to crème fraîche. Everyone makes this dip in their own way. On page 112, you'll find my personal favourite: a spicy guacamole with feta. In addition to guacamole, you can make lots of other tasty snacks with avocado. For example, there's the hummus-inspired avocado spread on page 106, and avocado bites with berbere – an Ethiopian spice mixture – which is always a hit at parties (see page 104).

118
SWEETS

In Europe it's still not common to use avocado in sweet dishes. In Brazil, on the other hand, they often do! Avocado is a wonderful alternative for cream and butter, so it's extremely well-suited for making vegan desserts. And avocado is ideal for people with a cow's milk allergy or lactose intolerance. In addition, it's also much healthier to incorporate a little fruit into your dessert instead of just dairy products and sugar. This chapter contains four different recipes – what do you think of these sweet variations on avocado?

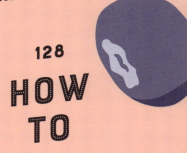

128
HOW
TO

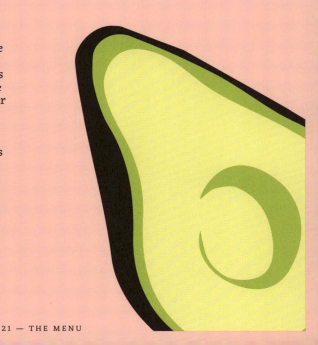

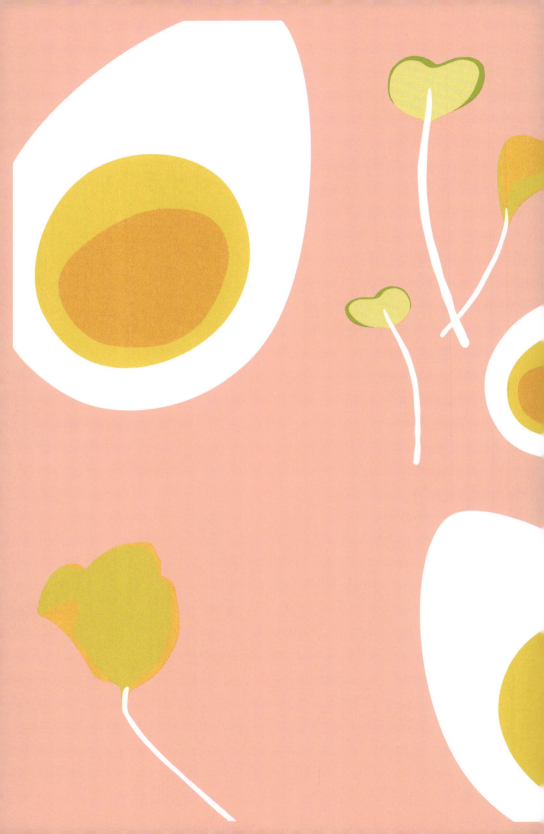

TOAST & EGGS

Extra love for your toast:
salmon, crispy bacon
or feta

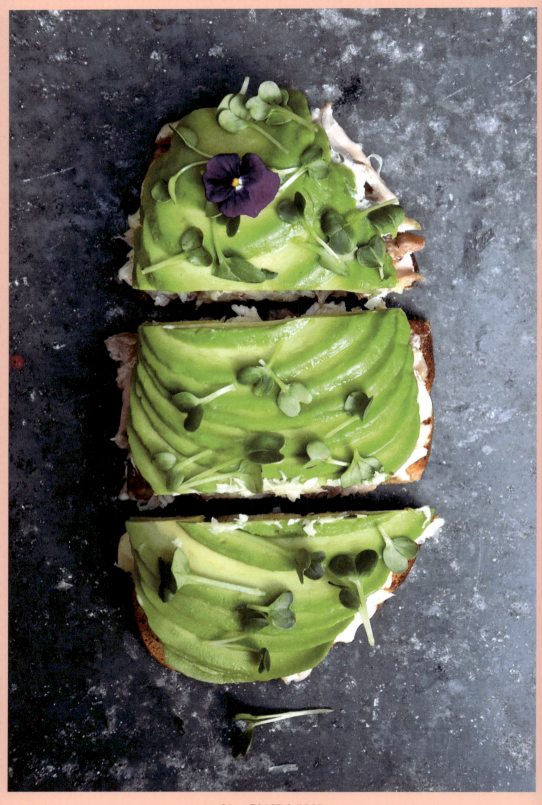

THE TRUFFLE TREASURE

Toast with avocado, chicken thighs, Parmesan cheese & 60-second homemade truffle mayo

Truffle combines beautifully with avocado, which is why this recipe also explains how to make a quick and easy truffle mayonnaise. Further along, you'll find another recipe that uses truffle mayonnaise: crispy gnocchi with avocado truffle bombs (see page 98).

Heat a large non-stick frying pan and add a little olive oil. Fry the chicken thigh fillets over high heat until golden brown and slightly crisp. Toast the slices of sourdough bread in a toaster.

Meanwhile, make the truffle mayonnaise. Pour the sunflower oil into a tall, narrow measuring jug (the one that came with your hand blender). Add all the mayonnaise ingredients, except for the egg yolk and the truffle tapenade. Gently place the egg yolk in the jug with the oil mixture. Jiggle the jug slightly so that the egg yolk is right in the middle on the bottom. Carefully place the hand blender over the egg yolk (don't break the yolk!) and switch it on. Very slowly (read: extremely slowly!) and in a single movement, pull up the hand blender until you've reached the surface of the emulsion. And voila: there's your mayonnaise!

Put the mayonnaise into a bowl and add the truffle tapenade. Use a little more tapenade if you're a big truffle fan. Taste and season with salt and pepper.

For the avocado fans, cut the avocado in half lengthwise, and remove the pit and the peel. Place both avocado halves (which you've rubbed with sushi vinegar) on your cutting board with the rounded side up, and cut them – crosswise – into thin slices. Gently press down on both halves to create a fan (allow the slices to overlap somewhat). When you're ready for them, use a flat (metal) spatula to transfer your fans.

Spread the truffle mayonnaise onto the hot toast. Use two forks to pull the chicken thigh fillets into shreds. Place the chicken on top of the truffle mayonnaise, sprinkle with the Parmesan cheese, and finish with the avocado fan, cress, pepper and salt.

When making the mayonnaise, it's absolutely essential that you do this in one single movement – if you stop, or move the hand blender back and forth, your mayonnaise will separate.

INGREDIENTS

olive oil

4 chicken thigh fillets (± 300g/10½oz)

2 thick slices of sourdough bread

1 avocado

sushi vinegar

2 tbsp truffle mayonnaise, homemade or shop-bought

30g/1oz Parmesan cheese, grated

cress

pepper and salt, to taste

FOR THE 60-SECOND HOMEMADE TRUFFLE MAYO

250ml/9fl oz/1 cup sunflower oil

juice of ½ a lemon

½ tsp white wine vinegar

1 tsp balsamic syrup

1 egg yolk, at room temperature

1 or 2 tbsp truffle tapenade

you will need: a hand blender

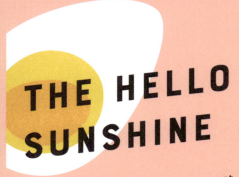

THE HELLO SUNSHINE

*Eggs sunny side up on crispy toast,
with edible flowers*

The perfect way to start your day

Cut the avocado in half lengthwise, and remove the pit and the peel. Rub both halves with a little sushi vinegar. This gives extra flavour and helps keep the avocado from discolouring.

Follow the steps for making an avocado rose on page 136 up to step 3. Once you've completed step 3, use the row of avocado slices to form a circle of approximately 10cm/4in in diameter. Do this twice.

Heat a large non-stick frying pan and add a little olive oil. Gently place the avocado circles in the pan, making sure that the bottom of the avocado fits snugly against the bottom of the pan so no egg white can escape while frying. Break the eggs into the avocado circles, and fry them till they're done to your satisfaction.

In the meantime, toast the bread in a toaster. With a spatula, carefully place the avocado suns onto the toast, and sprinkle with pepper and salt. If you like, you can decorate them with edible flowers and cress.

INGREDIENTS

1 avocado

sushi vinegar

(truffle) olive oil

2 eggs

2 slices of bread

pepper and salt, to taste

OPTIONAL

edible flowers and cress

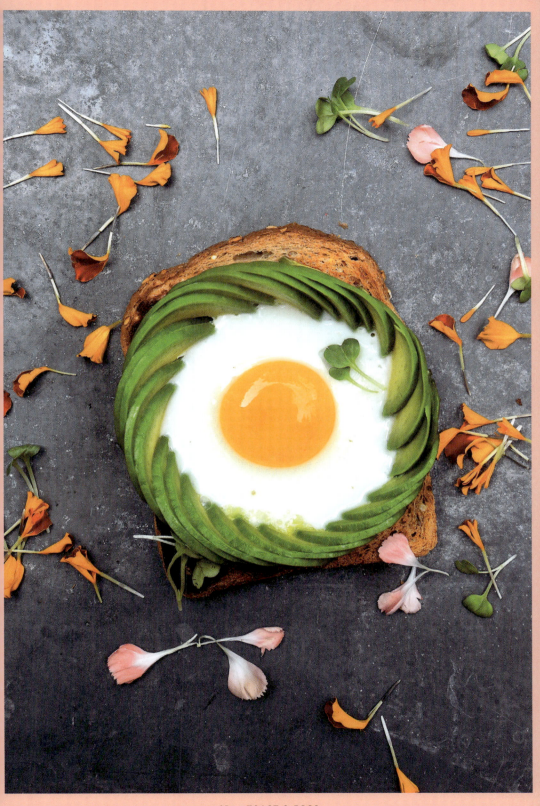

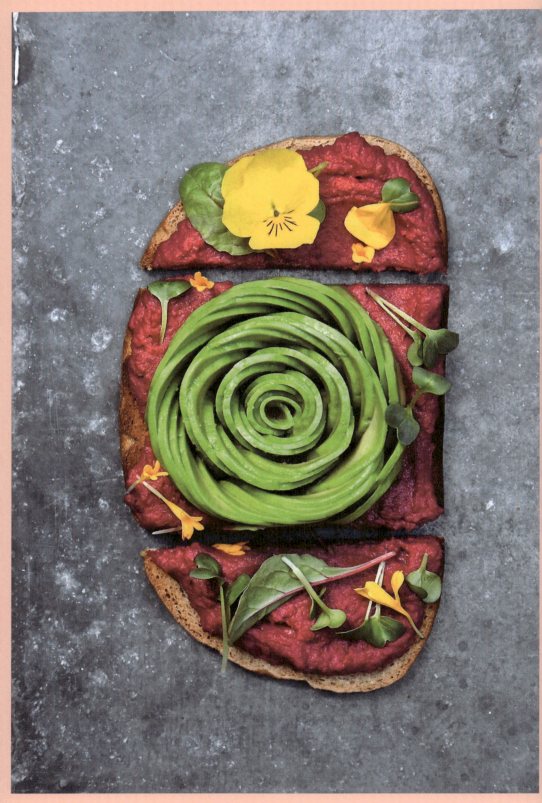

THE HEART-BEET ROSE

Red beetroot hummus on crispy toast, topped with an avocado rose

For the beetroot hummus, briefly blend the lemon juice, lemon zest, and garlic in a food processor. Add the cooked beetroot, chickpeas and tahini, and let the food processor run until everything is well blended. With the food processor running, slowly add first the cold water and then the olive oil and salt.

Make the avocado roses (see page 136). Toast the bread in a toaster or in a frying pan with a little olive oil. Spread the hummus onto the hot toast. Top each slice with an avocado rose and garnish with the toppings mentioned, or with whatever you think will be most delicious and beautiful.

— FETA —

ADD A LITTLE FETA TO THE HUMMUS, OR CRUMBLE SOME ONTO THE TOAST

INGREDIENTS

1 avocado

2 slices of bread

TOPPINGS

Swiss chard leaves, cress, and/or edible flowers (as pictured)

OPTIONAL

olive oil

FOR THE RED BEETROOT HUMMUS

juice of 1 lemon

the grated zest of ½ of an unsprayed lemon

1 garlic clove, grated

200g/7oz cooked red beetroot, cut into pieces

265g/9¼oz (drained weight) cooked chickpeas, drained

2 tbsp tahini (sesame seed paste)

2 tbsp cold water

2 tbsp olive oil

pinch of salt

you will need: a food processor

THE HOLY EGG & AVO

Avocado & egg-in-a-hole toast

An eggcelent choice in the morning

Preheat the oven to 200°C/400°F/gas 6.

Using a round cutter (8cm/3¼in in diameter), cut a circle out of one of the two bread slices. Brush both bread slices with (truffle) olive oil or spread them with salted butter. Cut the avocado in half, and remove the pit and the peel. Place the avocado half on your cutting board with the rounded side up. Cut the avocado half into three horizontally, and cut these pieces in half lengthwise. This will give you four (more or less) semicircles and two small pieces.

Stack the slices of bread on top of each other – the slice with the hole goes on top. Place the avocado semicircles inside the hole in two layers, fitting them up against the edge. Use the small pieces to fill gaps, where necessary. Place the sandwich on a baking sheet lined with baking parchment, and break the egg into the hole. Bake in the preheated oven, until the egg is done the way you like it. This will take about 20 minutes.

To serve as pictured: Cut the sandwich in half. In the photo, the two halves are stacked on top of each other. Add pepper, salt, chilli flakes, hot sauce, finely chopped spring onion (scallion), and/ or chives to taste.

— TIP —

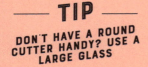

DON'T HAVE A ROUND CUTTER HANDY? USE A LARGE GLASS

INGREDIENTS

2 thick slices of bread (± 1.5cm/½in thick)

(truffle) olive oil or salted butter

½ an avocado

1 egg

pepper, salt, chilli flakes, hot sauce, spring onion (scallion) and/or chives, to taste

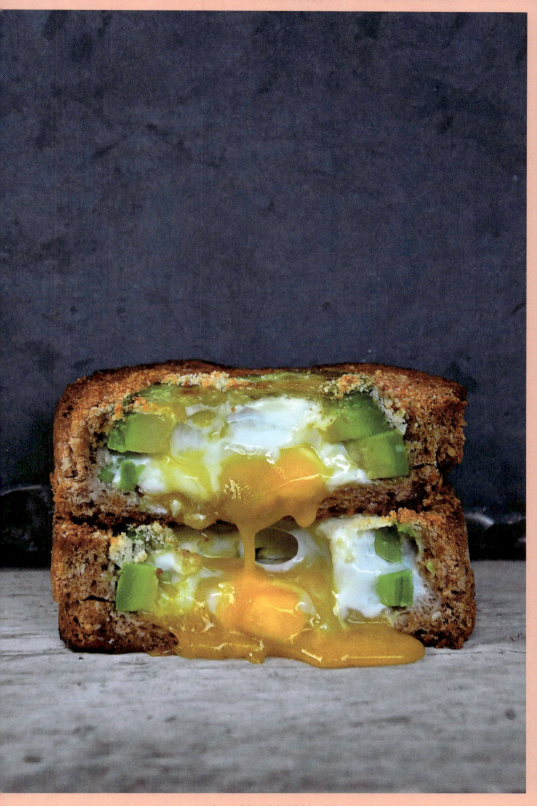

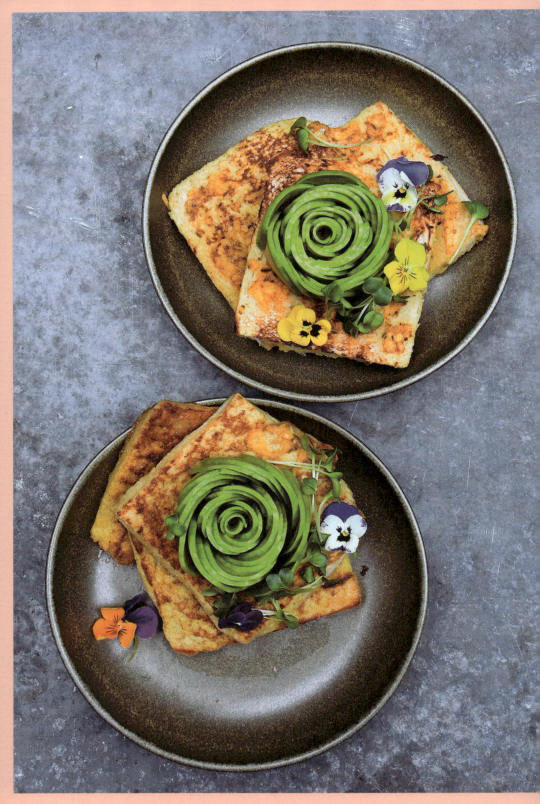

THE FRENCH TOAST

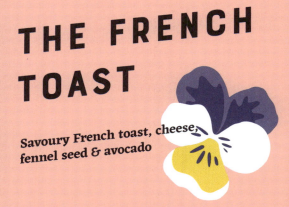

Savoury French toast, cheese, fennel seed & avocado

Are you as crazy about French toast as I am? Wouldn't it be nice to come up with an extra-special variation on this theme? Don't have a sweet tooth? Looking for a simple, kid-proof breakfast? This version is quick and easy to make – and you usually have all the necessary ingredients on hand. For a touch of decadence, add some crispy bacon or fry the French toast in truffle oil.

In a large bowl, whisk the eggs slightly. Add the milk, ground fennel seed and cheese to the eggs and mix well. Season with pepper and salt. Dip both sides of the bread into the mixture.

Heat a little olive oil or butter in a non-stick frying pan, and fry the French toast until crisp and golden brown.

Meanwhile, make two avocado roses (see page 136). Arrange the French toast on two plates. Top with an avocado rose, and serve with cress and edible flowers or watercress.

INGREDIENTS

2 eggs

100ml/3½fl oz/scant ½ cup milk

1 tbsp fennel seed, ground (use a pestle and mortar)

40g/1½oz grated (goat's) cheese

pepper and salt, to taste

6 small slices of (stale) white bread from a square sandwich loaf

olive oil or butter, for frying

1 avocado

sushi vinegar

TOPPINGS

cress, edible flowers, or watercress

optional (not pictured): chilli flakes

THE TOASTY TACO

With all of the goodness of tacos & avocados on toast

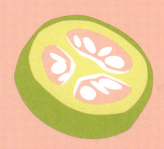

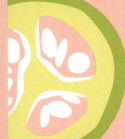

Although I could happily eat tacos every day, that might be taking things a bit too far. But if you're also a fan of the wonderful flavours and subtle heat, then give taco toast a try. You can make it as spicy as you like.

Make two avocado roses (see page 136). When you get to step 2, add alternate layers of thinly sliced Cheddar. Go on to the next step and finish the roses.

Toast the slices of sourdough bread in a toaster.

Spread the cream cheese on the hot toast, add a generous spoonful of tomato salsa, and – using a spatula – carefully add your avocado and Cheddar rose. Garnish your toast with all the toppings!

INGREDIENTS

1 avocado

sushi vinegar

60g/2oz Cheddar, thinly sliced (use a cheese slicer or vegetable peeler)

2 slices of sourdough bread

± 4 tbsp cream cheese

± 2 tbsp tomato salsa

TOPPINGS

½ a jalapeño pepper (use more or less to taste)

1 spring onion (scallion), finely chopped

1 sprig coriander (cilantro) (with stems), finely chopped

1 tsp grated lime zest

2 tbsp black beans, from a can

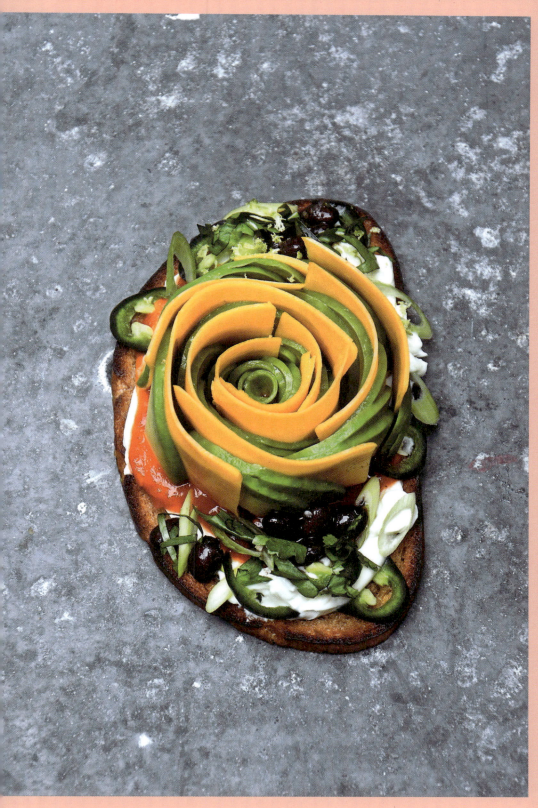

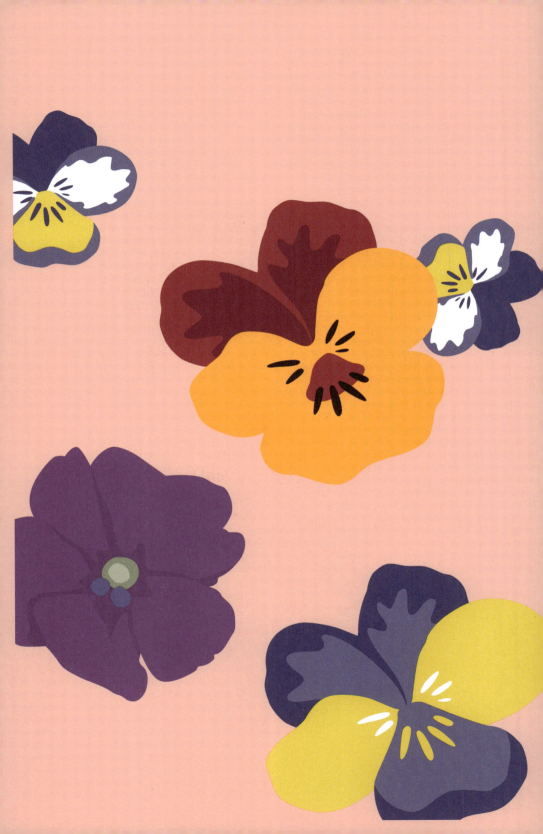

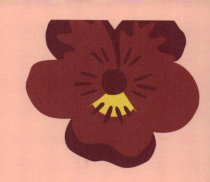

AVOCADO GARDENS

Hummus and avocado are a match made in heaven; it really is my favourite combination. For stylistic reasons – and maybe to some extent, for practical ones as well – I decided to serve the sauce, condiment, or dip in an avocado bowl. From soy sauce in avocado bowls (see Sushi Garden, page 44) to salad dressing in avocado bowls (see Balsamico Fantastico, page 58), the sky's the limit.

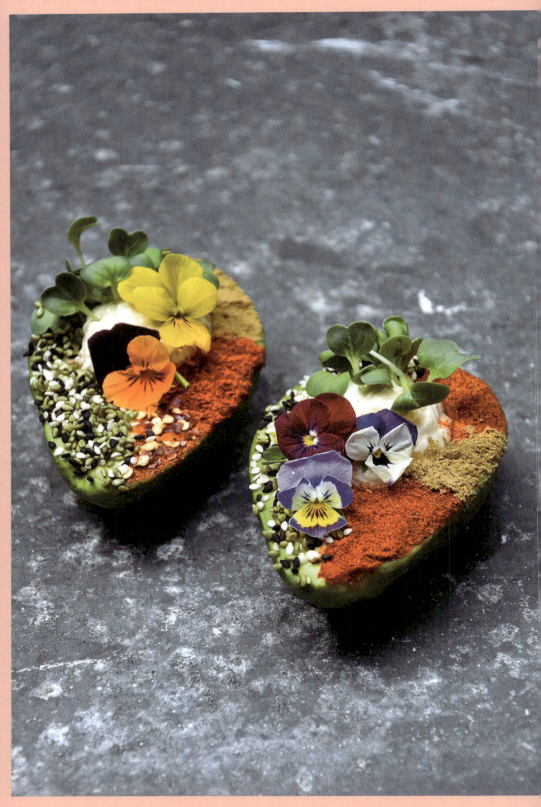

THE CLASSIC GARDEN

Avocado stuffed with hummus, spices, edible flowers & cress

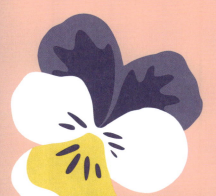

This is a real flavour bomb: it contains all the flavours that go beautifully with avocado! If you stick to this guideline for the right proportions of the various spices, I promise you can't go wrong.

Cut the avocado in half lengthwise, and remove the pit and the peel. Cut a small slice off the rounded side of both avocado halves so your avocado garden will be more stable.

Rub the avocado halves with sushi vinegar or a little lime juice. Fill both halves with hummus, and sprinkle the top rims of the avocado halves with sea salt to taste. To create well-defined sections, imagine that the top rim on the right side of the halves is divided into three sections. Dust with smoked paprika powder, ground cumin, cayenne pepper and/or chilli flakes. You can do this in any order you like, of course. Sprinkle the sesame seed mix on the top rim of the left side of the avocado halves. Carefully place a little cress in the centre of the hummus, and then decorate your garden with edible flowers.

INGREDIENTS

1 avocado

sushi vinegar or lime juice

2 tbsp hummus, homemade or your favourite shop-bought kind

sea salt, to taste

smoked paprika powder

ground cumin

cayenne pepper and/or chilli flakes

sesame seeds (a mixture of black, white, and green)

edible fresh and/or dried flowers

cress (daikon, basil, and/or Ghao)

crackers, a bagel, toast, or a fresh salad, to serve

THE GARDEN OF VEGAN

Avocado filled with lime & coriander hummus, gremolata, spices, sesame, edible flowers & cress

Coriander (cilantro): you either love it or you hate it! With coriander, you usually use both the leaves and the stems. For this hummus, you mainly use the stems; the leaves are perfect for decorating your garden. A classic hummus uses lemon juice, but for this coriander hummus, I use lime. It gives a delicious freshness to this garden!

For the hummus, process the chickpeas and the grated garlic in a food processor for a couple of minutes. Add the rest of the hummus ingredients – except for the salt – to the chickpea mixture, and process until well blended and smooth. Taste, and add salt if necessary.

In a small bowl, mix the ingredients for the gremolata. Taste, and season with pepper and salt.

Cut the avocado in half lengthwise, and remove the pit and the peel. Cut a small piece off the rounded side of both avocado halves so your avocado garden will be more stable on the plate.

Rub the avocado halves with sushi vinegar or lime juice. Fill both halves with hummus, and sprinkle the top rims of the avocado halves with sea salt to taste. Distribute the gremolata over the hummus, and top with cress and edible flowers. Decorate the tops of both halves with smoked paprika powder, black sesame seeds, and chilli flakes.

INGREDIENTS

1 avocado

sushi vinegar or lime juice

sea salt, to taste

cress

edible flowers

smoked paprika powder

black sesame seeds

chilli flakes

FOR THE LIME & CORIANDER HUMMUS

200g/7oz (drained weight) cooked chickpeas, drained

½ a small garlic clove, grated

juice and zest of 1 unsprayed lime

1 small bunch of coriander (cilantro), leaves and stems

2 generous tbsp tahini

salt, to taste

FOR THE GREMOLATA

zest of ½ an unsprayed lime

1 generous tbsp coriander leaves and stems, finely chopped

½ a small garlic clove, grated

pepper and salt, to taste

you will need: a food processor

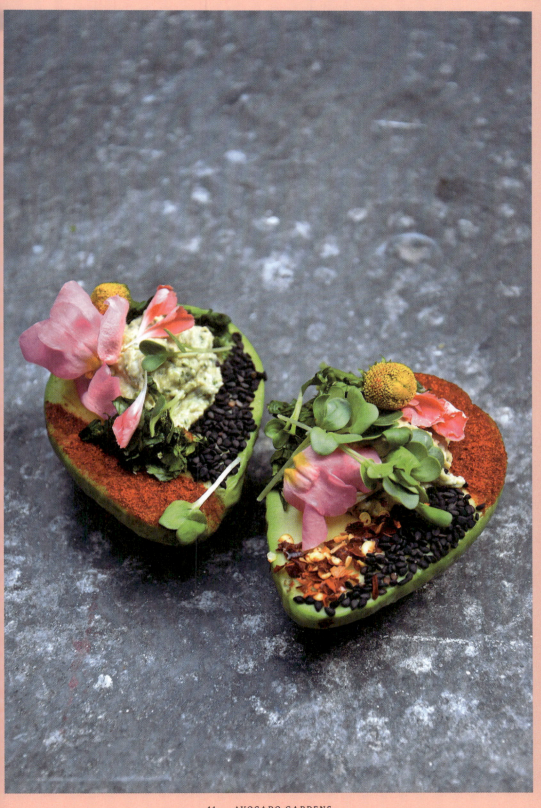

AVOCADO
A FRUIT.
A VEGETA
NOT A VE
BLE. NOT
VEGETAB

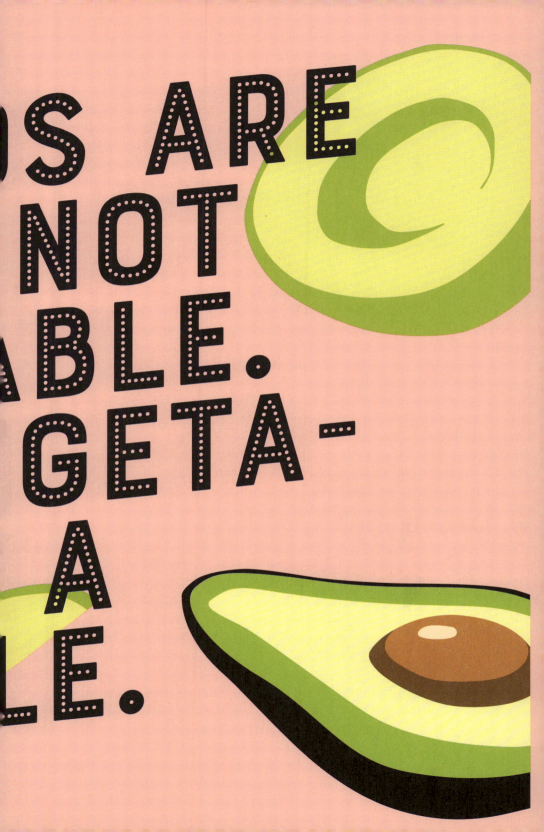

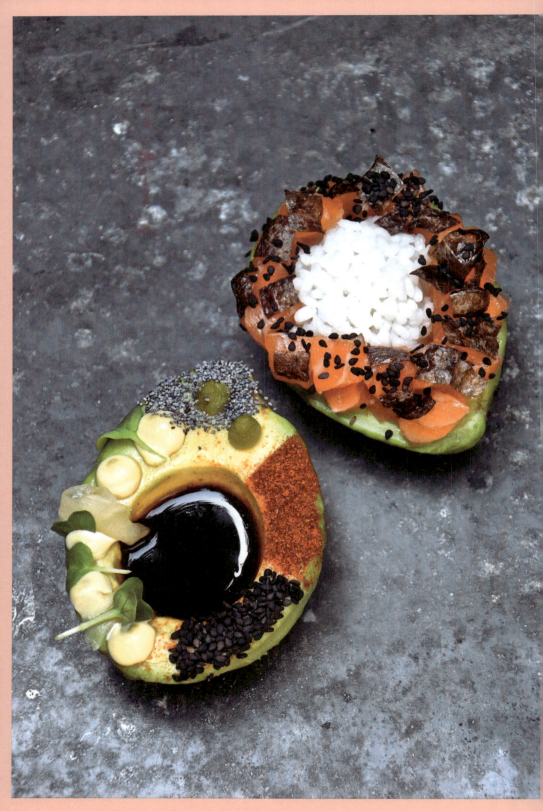

THE SUSHI GARDEN

Avocado stuffed with sushi rice, soy sauce, salmon, nori, pickled ginger, sesame seeds, poppy seeds, wasabi, spices & Japanese mayo

Cook the sushi rice according to the instructions on the packet.

Cut the avocados in half lengthwise, and remove the pit and the peel. Cut a small piece off the rounded side of all avocado halves so they will be more stable once they're on the plates. Rub all the halves with a little sushi vinegar.

Cut the salmon or tuna into small cubes. Place two avocado halves on each plate. On each plate, in the hollow left by the pit, fill one avocado half with soy sauce, and the other with sushi rice. Arrange the cubes of salmon or tuna, nori squares, and some black sesame seeds around the sushi rice. Decorate the surface around the soy sauce with dots of Japanese Kewpie mayonnaise, a little wasabi, pickled ginger, black sesame seeds, poppyseeds, cayenne pepper, and cress. Serve immediately.

For a vegetarian version, replace the fish with the marinated mango from page 52. For a vegan version, leave out the mayonnaise as well.

INGREDIENTS

100g/3½oz/scant ½ cup sushi rice

4 avocados

sushi vinegar

150g/5½oz fresh salmon or tuna (35g/1¼oz per person), sashimi quality

soy sauce

½ sheet of nori, cut into small squares with scissors

black sesame seeds

Japanese Kewpie mayonnaise

wasabi, to taste

pickled ginger, to taste

poppy seeds

cayenne pepper

cress

THE RAINBOW GARDEN

Avocado filled with beetroot hummus, spices, sesame seeds, edible flowers & cress

Cut the avocado in half lengthwise, and remove the pit and the peel. Cut a small piece off the rounded side of both avocado halves so they will be more stable once they're on the plate. Rub the avocado halves with the lime juice or sushi vinegar. Sprinkle the top surfaces of the avocado halves with sea salt to taste.

Create stripes in the colours of the rainbow, or in a variation on this theme, over the width of the avocado halves. Then fill the hollows left by the pit with the beetroot hummus. Garnish with cress and edible flowers.

Here's a really handy trick for making the coloured stripes: use bank cards. For the first stripe, place a card a generous 1cm/½in from the top of the avocado half. Dust with the smoked paprika powder. Then place the card a generous 1cm/½in below the red stripe. Hold another card over the red stripe, and sprinkle on the next colour. Continue in this way until you've dusted all the colours on. You can simply place the dried rose petals onto the avocado. Of course, the width of the stripes will depend on the size of your avocado. Instead of bank or other plastic cards, you can also use two strips of kitchen foil that have been folded in half.

INGREDIENTS

1 avocado

juice of a ¼ lime or a little sushi vinegar

sea salt, to taste

FOR THE

red stripe: smoked paprika powder

orange stripe: ground turmeric

yellow stripe: curry powder

green stripe: green sesame seeds (wasabi)

black stripe: black sesame seeds

pink stripe: dried rose petals

blue stripe: poppyseeds

2 generous tbsp beetroot hummus, your favourite shop-bought kind or home-made (see page 28)

TOPPINGS

cress (can also be used for the green stripe) and edible flowers

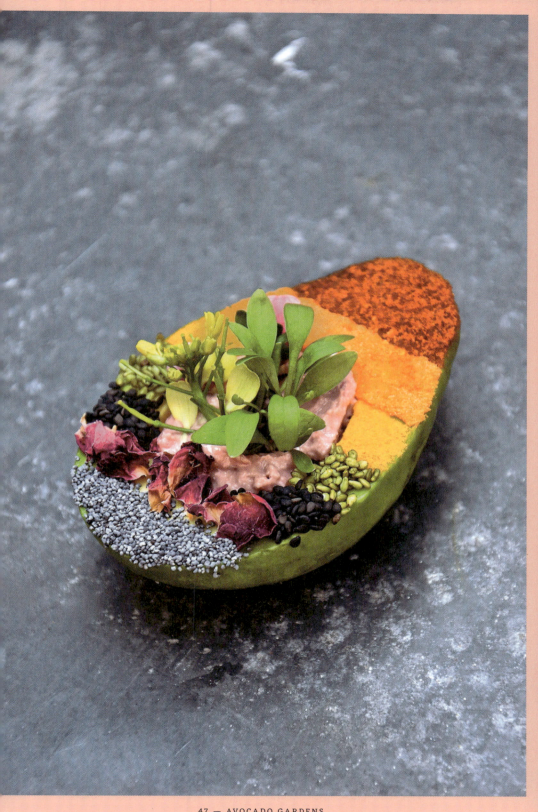

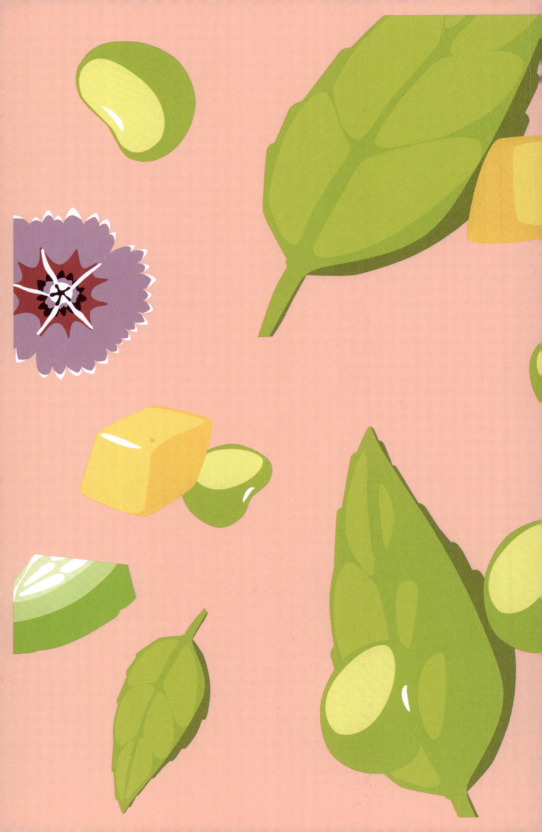

BOWLS & SALADS

These bowls and salads are packed with so much avocado goodness, you'll feel like a million bucks

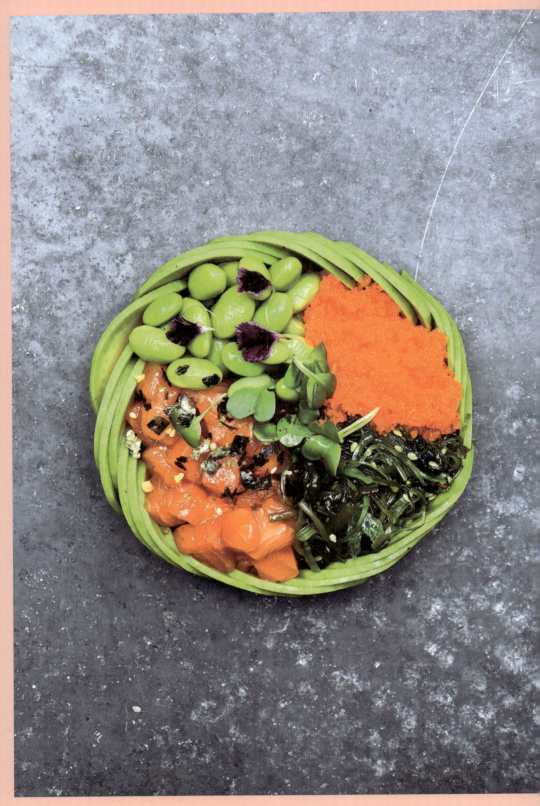

THE AVO POKE SHOW

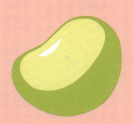

'Avocado bowl', sushi rice, raw salmon, wakame, edamame, tobiko roe & soy sauce

Cook the sushi rice according to the instructions on the packet.

Mix all the ingredients for the salmon marinade, cut the salmon into small cubes and add them to the marinade. Mix well to make sure all the salmon is coated with the marinade.

Make an avocado crown (see page 138). Fill the avocado crown – this will be the 'bowl' – with sushi rice. Press the rice down firmly with the back of a (wet) spoon.

On top of this, arrange the following ingredients: fill one quarter with salmon, one quarter with edamame beans, one quarter with tobiko fish roe, and one quarter with wakame salad. Sprinkle the furikake over the salmon, and arrange the flowers on top of the edamame. Place the cress in the middle of the poke bowl, and serve with soy sauce on the side.

— FURIKAKE —

FURIKAKE IS A DRY JAP-ANESE SEASONING THAT INCLUDES HORSERADISH, BONITO FLAKES, SESAME SEEDS, SEAWEED, AND DRIED VEGETABLES

INGREDIENTS

50g/1¾oz/scant ¼ cup sushi rice

± 50g/1¾oz salmon, sashimi quality

½ an avocado

2 tbsp edamame (soy) beans

2 tbsp tobiko fish roe

2 tbsp wakame seaweed salad

1 tbsp furikake (see Tip)

edible flowers, in a contrasting colour

daikon cress

soy sauce, to serve on the side

FOR THE SALMON MARINADE

½ tsp sushi vinegar

½ tsp soy sauce

1 tsp sesame oil

1 tsp olive oil

chilli flakes, to taste

THE VEGAN POKE SHOW

'Avocado bowl', sushi rice, mango, wakame, edamame, cucumber & soy sauce

Cook the sushi rice according to the instructions on the packet. Meanwhile, dice the cucumber and mix in the sushi vinegar.

Cube the mango, and marinate briefly in the chilli sauce with the black sesame seeds.

Make an avocado crown (see page 138). Fill the bowl with sushi rice. Press the rice down firmly with the back of a (wet) spoon.

On top of this, arrange the following ingredients: fill one quarter with mango, one quarter with cucumber, one quarter with edamame, and one quarter with wakame salad. Sprinkle some sesame seeds over the cucumber, and place the edible flowers on top of the edamame. Serve with soy sauce on the side.

INGREDIENTS

50g/1¾oz/scant ¼ cup sushi rice

½ a small cucumber

1 tsp sushi vinegar

¼ mango (± 100g/3½oz)

1 tsp chilli sauce

½ tsp black sesame seeds

½ an avocado

2 tbsp edamame (soy) beans

2 tbsp wakame seaweed salad

1 tsp sesame seeds

edible flowers

soy sauce, to serve on the side

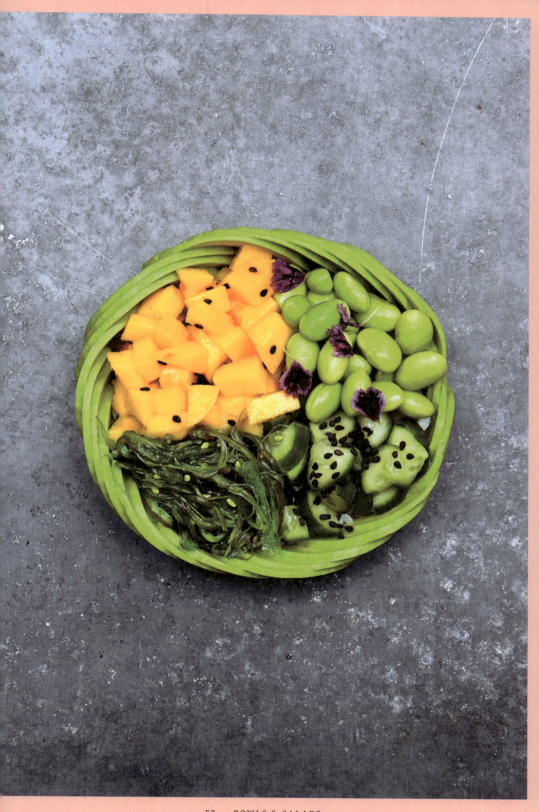

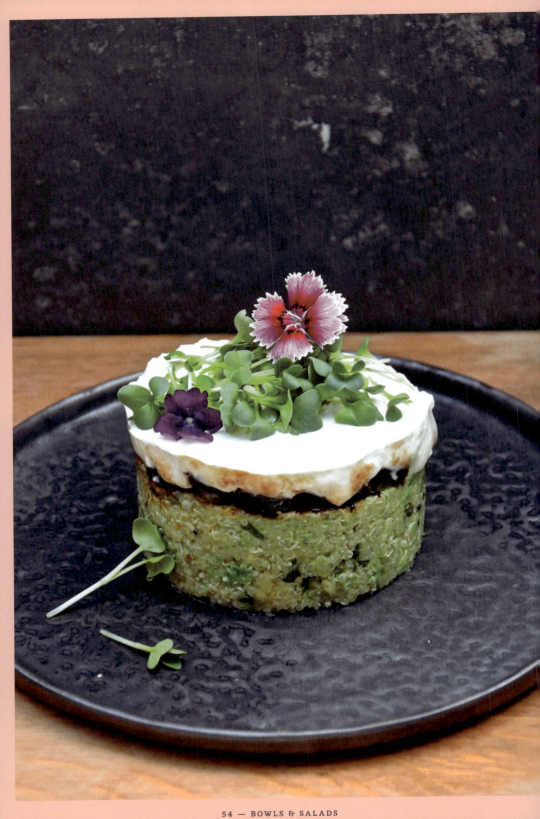

THE GUACINOA TOWER

Guacamole & quinoa tower with whipped feta & sticky balsamic onions

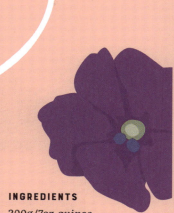

If you're worried the tower might collapse, you can always serve this salad in a bowl. But I assure you it will work – mixing the quinoa with the guacamole will give it extra body. Success guaranteed.

For the balsamic onions, mix the drained pickled onions with the balsamic vinegar and the brown sugar. Bring to the boil, then simmer over low heat for around 45 minutes until the liquid is reduced and the onions become sticky. Allow the onions to cool.

Meanwhile, prepare the quinoa according to the instructions on the packet and allow to cool. Cut the avocado in half lengthwise, and remove the pit and the peel. Scoop out the flesh into a bowl and coarsely mash it with a fork. Cut the lime in half, and squeeze the juice into the mashed avocado. Mix in the finely chopped coriander (cilantro), chilli flakes, spring onions (scallions) and garlic powder. Season with pepper and salt to taste. Add the quinoa to the guacamole and mix well.

Using a hand blender, blend the feta (or white cheese) with the water to make a nice whipped feta, which should be thick and creamy. Add extra water if necessary, but make sure the mixture remains thick.

Now start assembling the towers. Do this on the plate you'll be serving it on. Place the cutter in the middle of the plate. Spoon in a quarter of the guacamole–quinoa mixture, and press firmly. For the next layer, use a quarter of the sticky balsamic onions; distribute them evenly on top of the guacamole-quinoa mixture. End with a quarter of the whipped feta, and smooth off the top. Remove the cutter, and repeat for the other three plates. Garnish the towers with cress, chilli flakes to taste, and edible flowers.

— TIP —

ALSO DELICIOUS: SUBSTI-TUTE CAULIFLOWER RICE FOR QUINOA

INGREDIENTS

200g/7oz quinoa

2 avocados

1 lime

a bunch of fresh coriander (cilantro), finely chopped

1 tsp chilli flakes (+ extra for serving)

2 spring onions (scallions), finely chopped

1 tsp garlic powder

pepper and salt, to taste

200g/7oz feta (or white cheese)

75ml/2½fl oz/5 tbsp water

FOR THE BALSAMIC ONIONS

190g/6¾oz (drained weight) pickled cocktail onions

150ml/5fl oz/scant ⅔ cup balsamic vinegar

1 tsp brown sugar

OPTIONAL

cress and edible flowers

you will need: a tall cutter

THE KING KALE BOWL

Crunchy kale salad & avocado roses

Kale lends itself perfectly to this vibrant and nutritious salad. The acid and oil in the vinaigrette, combined with a brief massage, results in a deliciously tender marinated kale salad. You only have to knead the salad for a minute (don't squeeze) – the kale will wilt, and beautifully absorb all the amazing flavours.

Stir together the olive oil, lemon juice, and grated garlic to make a nice vinaigrette. Add pepper and salt to taste.

Put the kale, Parmesan cheese, and smoked almonds into a large bowl. Pour over the vinaigrette. With your hands, knead the salad well for about a minute.

Make four avocado roses (see page 136), rubbing the avocados with sushi vinegar to keep them from discolouring. Spoon the salad into four dishes, and top the salads with the roses. Serve with extra Parmesan cheese and almonds.

— HOW TO —

THERE'S ALSO A PIXELATED AVOCADO IN THE PHOTO. CHECK PAGE 140 FOR INSTRUCTIONS ON HOW TO MAKE THIS

INGREDIENTS

100ml/3½fl oz/scant ½ cup olive oil

juice of 1 lemon

1 small or ⅓ a large garlic clove, grated

pepper and salt, to taste

200g/7oz kale, chopped

40g/1½oz Parmesan cheese, finely grated (+ extra for serving)

± 75g/2½oz/heaped ½ cup smoked almonds, roughly chopped (+ extra, for serving)

2 avocados

sushi vinegar

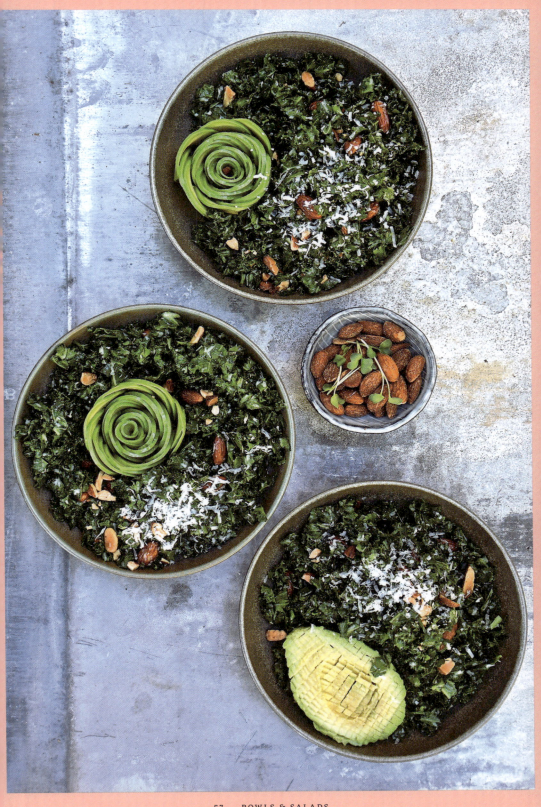

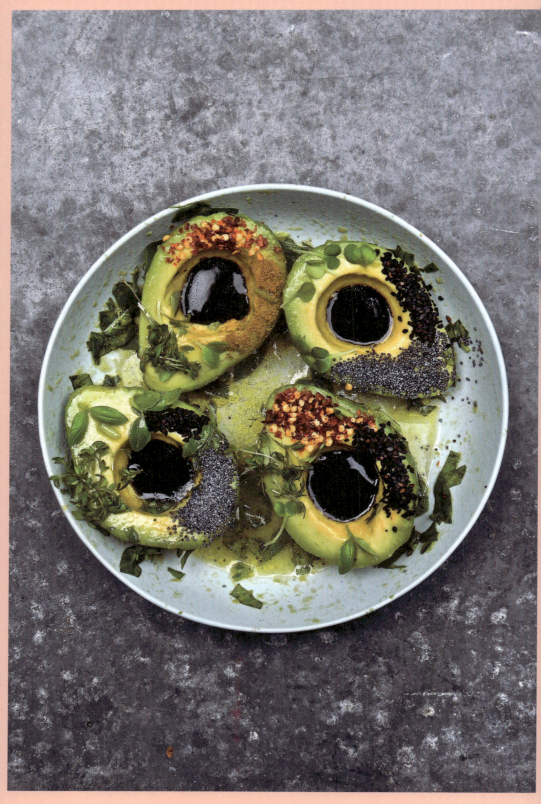

THE BALSAMICO FANTASTICO

Marinated avocado & balsamic syrup

These marinated avocados are wonderful as a starting point for a salad or as a side dish for a BBQ. They're deliciously tangy, for a nice 'bite'. If you'd like yours to be a little less tart, use the juice of half a lemon.

In a small dish (but large enough to fit four avocado halves), mix together the lemon zest, lemon juice, and olive oil. Add salt to taste. Finely chop the basil, and stir it in.

Cut the avocados in half lengthwise, and remove the pit and the peel. Place the avocados in the dish. Rub the marinade thoroughly onto all sides of the avocado halves. Cover the dish, and refrigerate for at least 20 minutes; a couple of hours is also fine. Don't worry, the acid in the lemons will keep the avocados nice and green.

Take the avocados out of the fridge. Decorate with your choice of toppings, and pour balsamic syrup into the hollows left by the pit.

INGREDIENTS

grated zest of ½ a small unsprayed lemon

juice of 1 small lemon

4 tbsp olive oil

pinch of sea salt

a small bunch of basil (+ extra for serving)

2 avocados

balsamic syrup

— UPGRADE —
DELICIOUS SERVED WITH A GOAT'S CHEESE SALAD

TOPPINGS

chilli flakes, poppyseeds, sesame seeds, ground cumin, cress, and basil

THE PRETTY SWEET POTATO

Loaded sweet potato with mozzarella, pesto & avocado

A generous helping of fruit (avocado) and vegetables (sweet potato), and also a great combination of flavours, textures and temperatures. Perfect for #meatlessmonday

Preheat the oven to 200°C/400°F/gas 6. Bake the unpeeled sweet potatoes in a baking dish until tender. This will take about 45 to 60 minutes, depending on the size of the sweet potatoes. Also, every oven is different.

Meanwhile, make the pesto. First, mix the basil, olive oil, and the garlic in a food processor. Add the cheese and process briefly. Finally, add the cashews, and process the pesto until it's as chunky or as smooth as you like. If necessary, add a little extra olive oil until the pesto is rich and creamy. Add pepper and salt to taste.

Dice the tomatoes and make four avocado roses (see page 136). Take the sweet potatoes out of the oven and cut them open down the middle. Fill the sweet potatoes with the mozzarella, tomato, and pesto. Top with the avocado roses.

— **CHEESE!** —

NOT A BIG MOZZAREL-LA FAN? USE FETA OR GOAT'S CHEESE

INGREDIENTS

4 sweet potatoes, unpeeled

2 tomatoes

2 avocados

1 ball of buffalo mozzarella, torn into pieces

OPTIONAL

cress or basil leaves

FOR THE PESTO

1 large bunch of basil, thick stems removed

3½ tbsp good-quality olive oil (+ extra, if neccesary)

1 small garlic clove, grated

50g/1¾oz aged cheese, grated

50g/1¾oz cashews

pepper and salt

you will need: a food processor

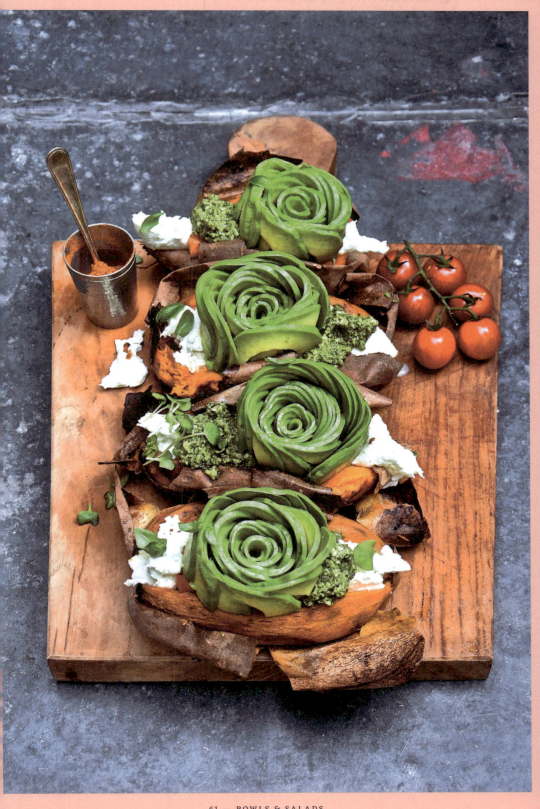

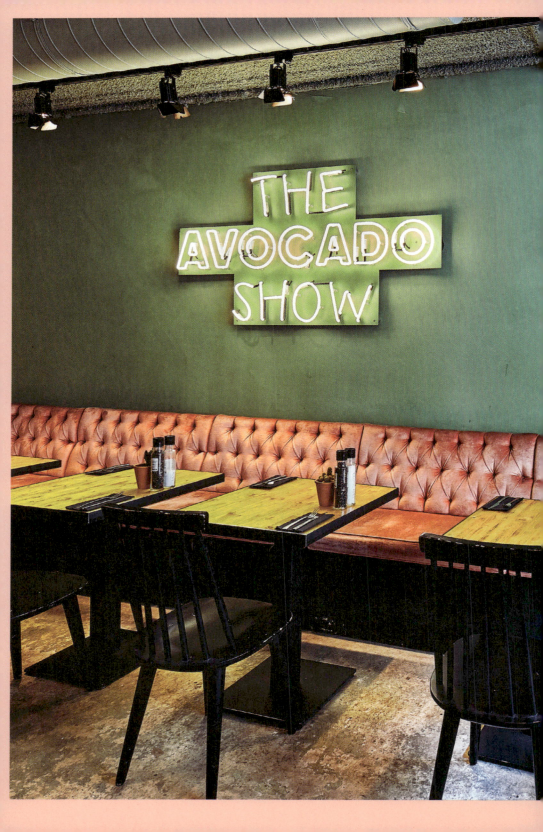

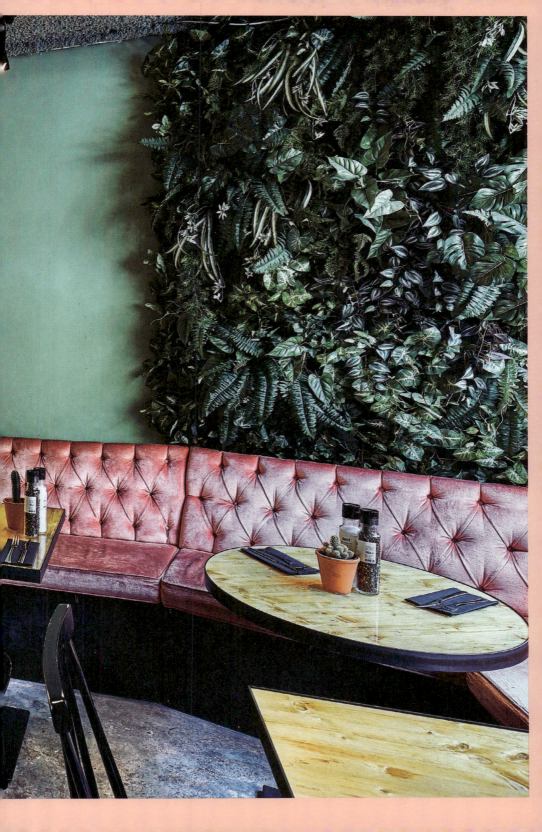

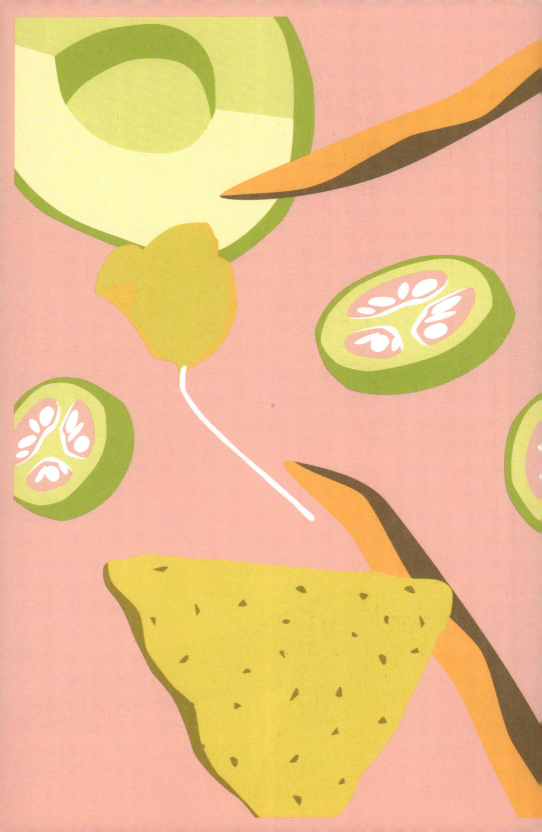

FANCY FAST FOOD

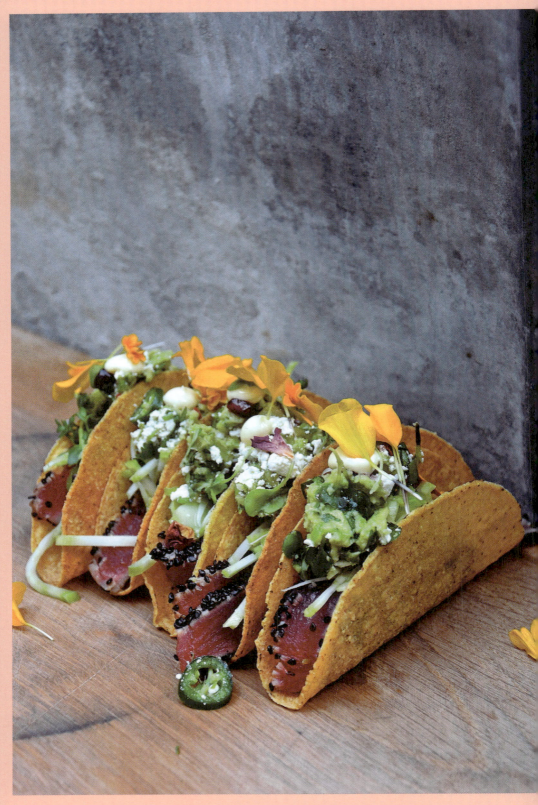

THE TUNA TATACO

Crispy taco, tuna tataki, broccoli, spicy guacamole & Japanese mayo

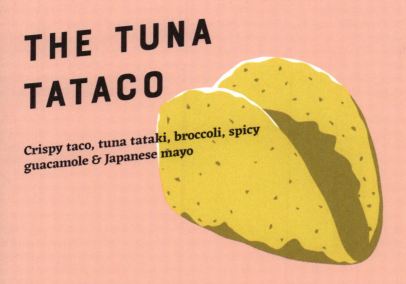

This is one of those dishes that comes into being when you're 'cooking with whatever you've got to hand'. It just so happened I'd scored some beautiful fresh tuna that day, but hadn't yet decided what I was going to make with it. Then a package of hard-shell tacos caught my eye, and this recipe was the result.

Preheat the oven to 180°C/350ºF/gas 4.

With a sharp knife, cut the broccoli stems into julienne (strips the size of matchsticks). Mix the strips with the truffle oil and add salt to taste.

Make The Fooddeco Spicy Feta on page 112. Skip the step for making the avocado rose, and instead mash everything into guacamole straight away.

Coat the tuna with the black sesame seeds, and sear it lightly (on both sides) in a red-hot grill pan. A frying pan will also work. Cut the tuna into thin slices. You now have tuna tataki.

Place the taco shells in the preheated oven, and heat for the length of time given on the box. Fill the hot taco shells with the tuna tataki, broccoli salad and guacamole (don't use it all!). Finish with dots of Japanese mayonnaise, cress and edible flowers. Serve immediately, along with the leftover guacamole (in an attractive dish).

— TIP —

INSTEAD OF TUNA, YOU CAN USE SALMON OR STEAK

INGREDIENTS

80g/2¾oz broccoli stems

1 tbsp truffle oil

salt, to taste

The Fooddeco Spicy Feta guacamole (see page 112), with everything coarsely mashed at the start

200g/7oz raw tuna, sashimi quality

black sesame seeds

6 hard-shell tacos

Japanese Kewpie mayonnaise

TOPPINGS

cress, edible flowers and pomegranate seeds

THE AVO NUGGETS

Crunchy avocado nuggets, almonds, crispy fried onions, sesame seeds & honey-mustard sauce

Chicken nuggets are one of the most popular fast food snacks. There's no deep fat fryer involved when it comes to these avocado nuggets, which are made from raw avocado with a crunchy layer of crispy fried onions, nuts and sesame seeds.

In a dry frying pan, toast the flaked almonds until golden brown. Spoon the almonds into a container or bowl and allow to cool. Meanwhile, cut the avocado in half lengthwise, and remove the pit and the peel. Cut both avocado halves into three lengthwise, and then into three crosswise. You will now have nine pieces per half. Rub them with the lime juice or sushi vinegar. Make the honey-mustard sauce by stirring together all of the sauce ingredients.

Add the crispy fried onions and the sesame seeds to the flaked almonds and mix well. Roll the pieces of avocado through this mixture one at a time, using a little bit of pressure to make sure the mixture sticks well. Eat at once, while they're still nice and crunchy, with the honey–mustard sauce alongside.

— TIP —

TRY SERVING THEM IN AN OLD LOAF TIN LINED WITH BAKING PARCHMENT

INGREDIENTS

4 tbsp flaked almonds

1 avocado

juice of a ¼ lime or a little sushi vinegar

4 tbsp crispy fried onions (ready-made)

4 tbsp sesame seeds

FOR THE HONEY-MUSTARD SAUCE

1 tbsp mayonnaise

1 tbsp yellow mustard

1 tbsp honey

salt, to taste

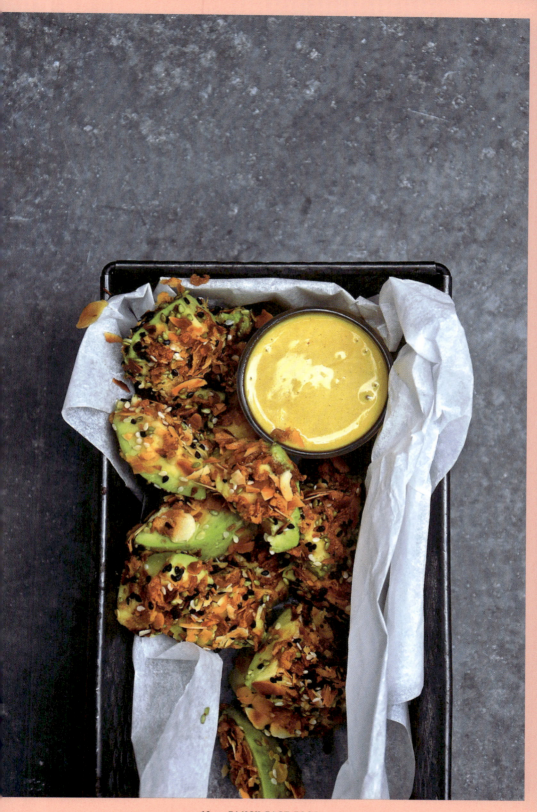

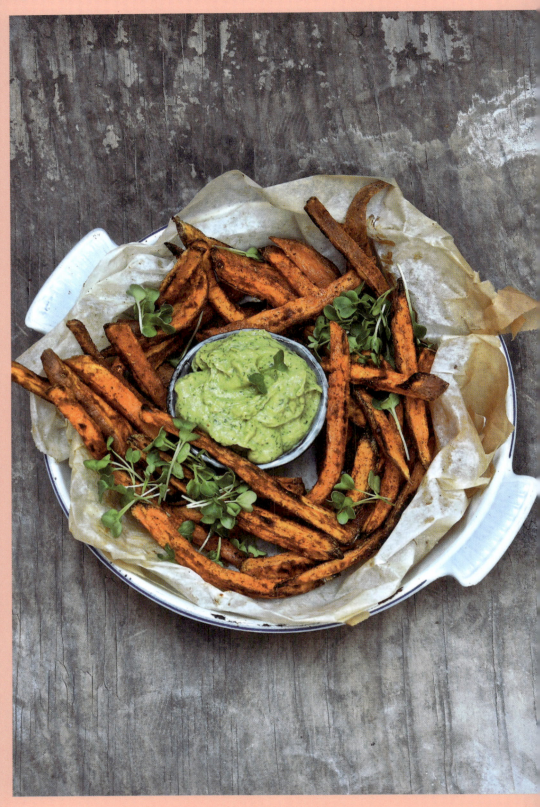

THE FRIES BEFORE GUYS SAUCE

Fooddeco's legendary avocado frites sauce

You can make an incredible *frites* sauce with just three ingredients. It's mayo-free, so vegans can also dip away, as much as they like. You can serve this sauce as pictured, with homemade sweet potato chips (fries). But it's also delicious with oven chips or fried potatoes (the secret is to flip them one at a time). Or nice and easy: get some takeaway chips.

Pan-fry, deep-fry, or bake your favourite chips or potatoes.

To make the sauce, cut the avocado in half lengthwise, remove the pit, and scoop out the flesh into a bowl. Add the dill and the piccalilli. Puree the mixture with a hand blender until completely smooth, but make sure you can still see some dill. Taste, and add salt if necessary.

Serve with the *frites* sauce.

To style this dish as pictured, put the chips – baking parchment and all – in an attractive (not overly large) baking dish. Tuck in a small bowl of the *frites* sauce, and garnish with some cress, rocket (arugula) or fresh herbs.

INGREDIENTS

sweet potato chips (home-made, or your favourite shop-bought kind)

1 avocado

2 tbsp fresh dill, finely chopped (± 10g/⅓oz)

3 tbsp piccalilli

salt

TOPPINGS

cress, rocket (arugula) and/ or fresh herbs

you will need: a hand blender

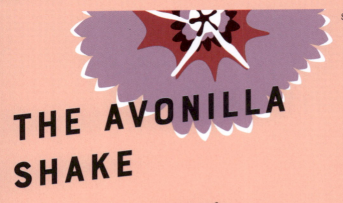

THE AVONILLA SHAKE

**Avocado-banana-vanilla milkshake
& a chocolate rim 'how-to'**

This ice-cold creamy beverage is sublime on a hot summer day. At our house, it also often features as a breakfast item throughout the year.

Melt the chocolate in a bain-marie. Turn a glass (or jar) upside-down and spoon a generous amount of chocolate along the upper rim of the glass. Rotate the glass until you've coated the entire rim. Now turn the glass right side up, and the chocolate will run down the sides. Make sure you're close to the freezer. If you're happy with the chocolate pattern, put the glass in the freezer at once, and leave it there for at least 5 minutes. Repeat with the second glass.

Meanwhile, make the milkshake. Blend all the ingredients in a food processor until smooth. Pour the milkshake into the glasses (or jars), and add straws. Serve immediately.

GLASS

I ALWAYS SERVE THIS IN JARS, BUT YOU CAN ALSO USE STURDY GLASSES

INGREDIENTS

1 frozen banana, sliced (put it in the freezer the night before)

flesh of 1 avocado

100ml/3½fl oz/scant ½ cup (coconut) yoghurt

100ml/3½fl oz/scant ½ cup almond milk, unsweetened

1 tbsp honey

1 or 2 tsp vanilla extract

FOR THE CHOCOLATE RIM

50g/1¾oz dark chocolate (70% cocoa solids)

you will need: a food processor

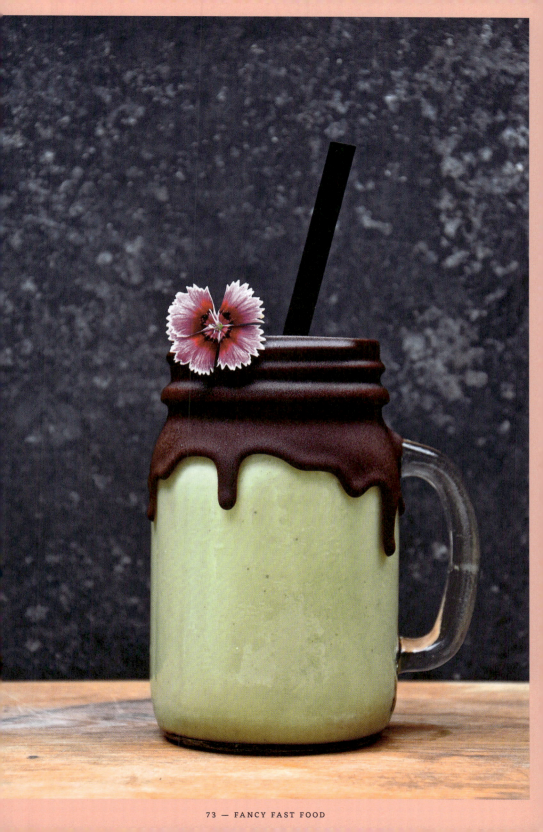

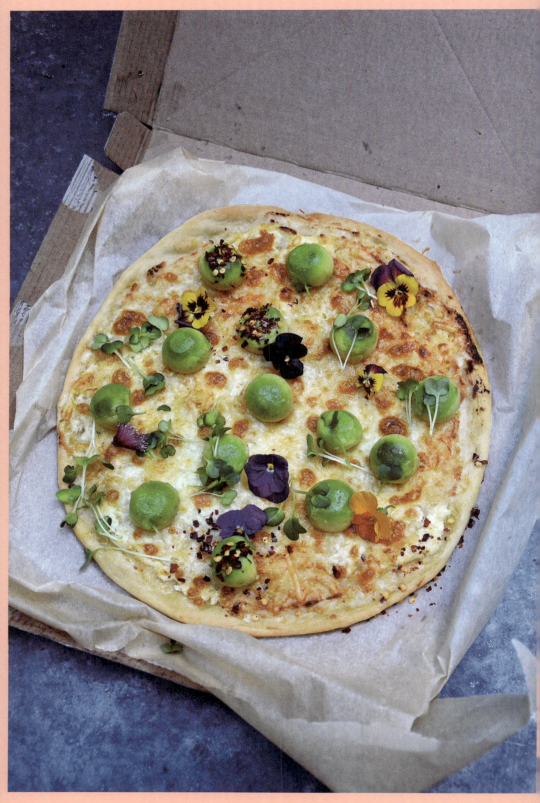

THE PIZZA BIANCA

Pizza with avocado pepperoni

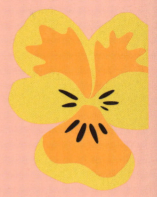

Pepperoni is a spicy salami. On this pizza, the pepperoni slices are replaced by spicy avocado balls. Use chilli flakes to make the 'avocado pepperoni' as spicy as you like.

First, make the dough. Dissolve the yeast in 50ml/1¾fl oz/3½ tbsp lukewarm water. Place the flour in a large mixing bowl and make a deep well in the centre. Sprinkle the salt over the flour. Now pour in the yeast mixture, the remaining lukewarm water, and a tablespoon of olive oil. Slowly stir the liquids in the well with a fork or spoon, gradually adding in more of the flour from the sides until everything is well mixed. Vigorously knead the dough for another 15 minutes: push, pull, and knead it in the bowl until it forms a firm ball that is no longer sticky. Take the dough ball out, pour a teaspoon of olive oil into the bowl, add back the ball, and roll it around in the oil. Cover with a damp tea towel. Allow the dough to rise in a warm place for 2 hours.

Preheat the oven to 220°C/425ºF/gas 7.

Divide the dough into two balls. On baking parchment, roll them out to form two thin pizza bases of around 26cm/10⅓in in diameter. Mix the olive oil with the garlic, and spread it onto both of the bases, leaving the edge (around 1cm/½in) of the pizza base uncoated for the crust. Spread the bases with the ricotta or cream cheese. Tear the mozzarella into pieces and distribute evenly over both bases, then grate on the Parmesan cheese. Sprinkle the pizzas with the Gouda cheese. Bake in the oven for about 15 minutes until golden brown.

Meanwhile, cut the avocado in half lengthwise, and remove the pit and the peel. Rub both halves with sushi vinegar. Now use the melon baller to make the avocado balls. Take the pizza out of the oven, add the avocado pepperoni, and sprinkle with chilli flakes to taste. Garnish the pizza with cress and edible flowers.

No time to make pizza dough from scratch? You'll find plenty of ready-made doughs and pizza bases in the supermarket.

INGREDIENTS

2 tbsp olive oil

1 garlic clove, grated

2 generous tbsp ricotta or cream cheese

1 mozzarella ball (± 125g/4½oz)

40g/1½oz Parmesan cheese

40g/1½oz Gouda cheese, grated

1 avocado

sushi vinegar

chilli flakes

FOR THE DOUGH

7g/¼oz yeast

150ml/5fl oz/scant ⅔ cup lukewarm water

250g/9oz/heaped 1¾ cups 00 (fine) flour, suitable for pizza dough

1 tsp salt

1 tbsp olive oil (+ 1 tsp extra)

TOPPINGS

edible violets and cress

you will need: a melon baller

THE AVO SATÉ

Loaded avocado satay skewers

How about *alpukat* satay for a change, instead of *ayam* (chicken), *babi* (pork) or *Padang*?

Cut the avocados in half lengthwise, and remove the pits and the peel. Rub the avocado halves with lime juice or sushi vinegar. Cut them into three lengthwise, and then into three crosswise. You now have nine avocado chunks per avocado half; they don't all need to be the same size. Thread them onto the wooden skewers and place them on a platter. Cover the platter and put it into the fridge.

Meanwhile, prepare the peanut sauce. Finely chop the spring onion (scallion) and the coriander (cilantro), and slice the red chilli into small rings.

When the peanut sauce is ready, take the skewers out of the fridge. Sprinkle the smoked paprika powder over the avocado satay skewers, and pour on some of the peanut sauce. Add the red chilli rings (to taste), finely chopped coriander, crispy fried onions, spring onions, peanuts, and also daikon cress if desired. Pour the rest of the peanut sauce into a pretty dish to serve on the side.

INGREDIENTS

4 avocados

juice of ½ a lime or a little sushi vinegar

400ml/14fl oz/1¾ cups Indonesian peanut sauce (satay sauce), homemade or your favourite shop-bought kind

1 spring onion (scallion)

1 small bunch of coriander (cilantro), including the stems

1 red chilli pepper

1 tsp smoked paprika powder

crispy fried onions (ready-made)

a handful of peanuts

OPTIONAL

daikon cress

you will need: (wooden) skewers or lollipop sticks (ice cream sticks)

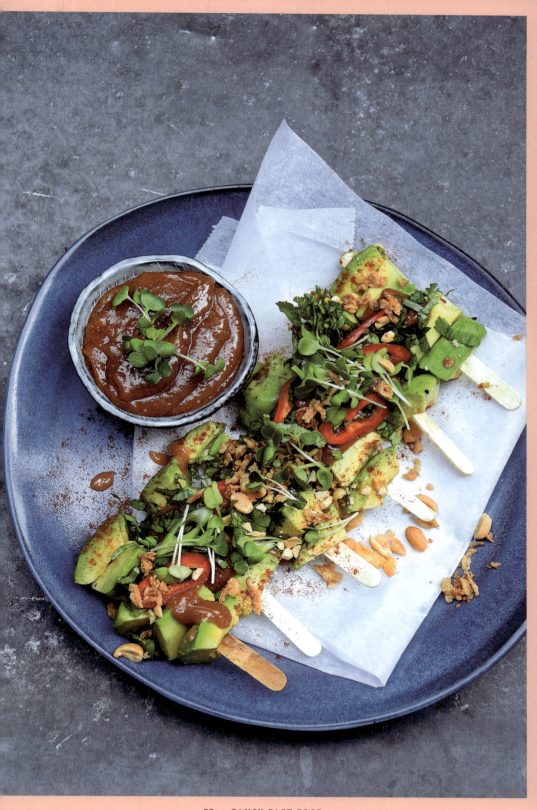

THE CARROT DOG

Smoky carrot hot dog

The marinade gives the carrot a smoky sausage-like flavour. You'll need to be a little patient, because the carrots need to marinate overnight. Combining the carrot dog with the flavours of a classic hot dog (mustard, pickle, onions and ketchup) gives you the flavour palette of a real hot dog, but in a vegan version. Serve it all in an avocado bun.

Peel the carrots with a vegetable peeler, and round off both ends so they resemble a hot dog. Cook the carrots for 10 to 15 minutes until quite tender.

Meanwhile, mix together all the marinade ingredients in a saucepan (preferably large enough to fit the hot dog carrots) and bring to a boil. Add the carrots to the marinade, and turn off the heat. Allow to cool, then put the carrots along with the marinade into a plastic (ziplock) bag. Refrigerate for at least 4 hours, but preferably overnight. To avoid accidents, it's a good idea to place the bag on a deep plate.

Make avocado buns as described on page 139, with one exception: cut the buns in half lengthwise, not crosswise. Squeeze some ketchup into the hollows left by the pits. Take the carrot dogs out of the marinade. If you like, you can also heat them briefly in a frying pan. Place them on the four bottom halves of the avocados.

Add your choice of toppings, then add the upper halves of the avocados, and garnish the tops of the avocado buns with sesame seeds to make them look like real ones.

Serve the hot dog in a small basket lined with baking parchment, along with extra toppings.

SAUSAGE

YOU CAN, OF COURSE, ALSO MAKE THIS AVOCADO BUN WITH A REAL HOT DOG

INGREDIENTS

4 carrots, about the size of a hot dog

4 avocados

FOR THE MARINADE

50ml/1¾fl oz/3½ tbsp soy sauce

50ml/1¾fl oz/3½ tbsp vegetable stock

2 tbsp ginger syrup (for example, from a jar of stem ginger)

2 tbsp sushi vinegar

1 tsp smoked paprika powder

1 tsp yellow mustard

TOPPINGS

ketchup, yellow mustard, crispy fried onions, red onion (finely chopped), gherkins, and sesame seeds

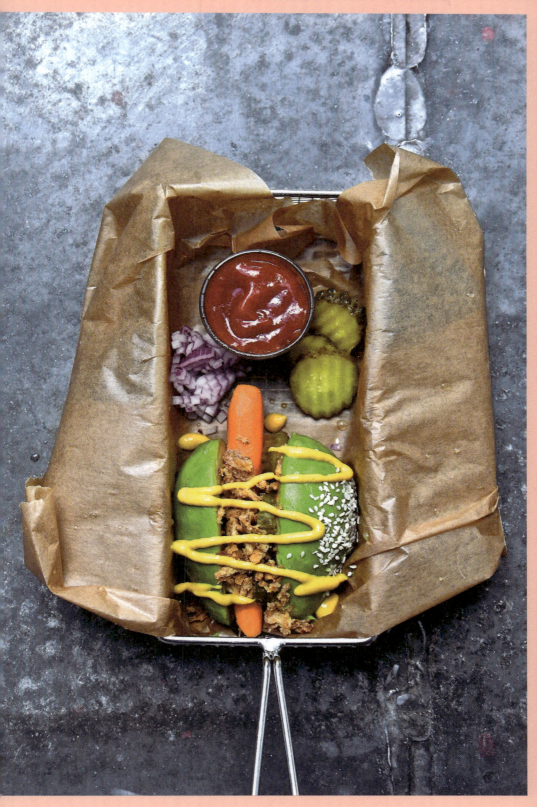

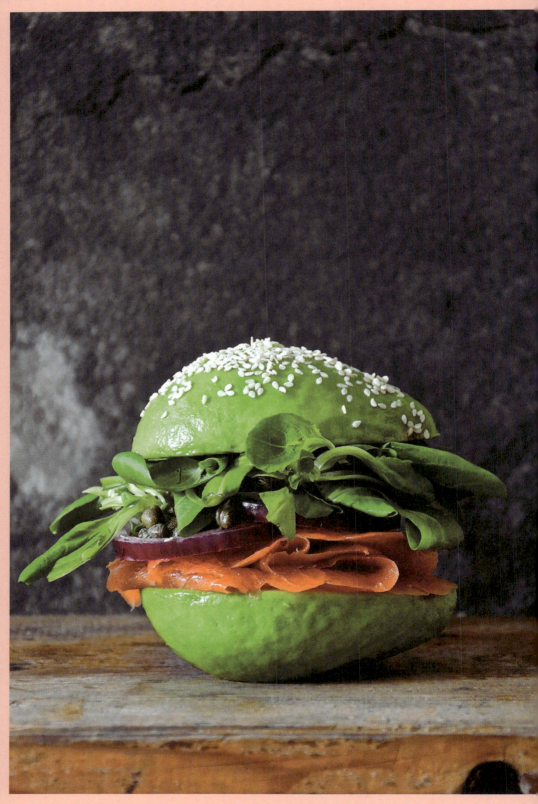

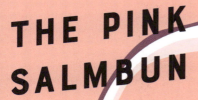

THE PINK SALMBUN

Smoked salmon sandwich & remoulade

This is a type of stacked salad, and you can serve it with toast or a warm bagel. Remoulade is traditionally eaten with fried fish, but avocado goes really well with it: the combination of remoulade and creamy avocado is incredibly good.

In a bowl, mix together all the ingredients for the remoulade sauce, except for the egg. Peel the egg, and with the back of a spoon, push the egg through a fine sieve over the sauce. Stir well and season with pepper and salt. Cover and put in the fridge for at least 20 minutes, so the flavours can meld.

Make avocado buns as described on page 139, with one exception: cut the buns in half lengthwise, not crosswise. Rub the avocado halves with sushi vinegar.

Fill the bottom halves – in the hollow that held the pit – with remoulade sauce. On top of this, arrange the smoked salmon, lamb's lettuce, sliced red onion, and capers. Now add the upper halves of the avocados, and garnish the tops of the avocado buns with sesame seeds to make them look like real sesame seed buns. Insert a wooden skewer into the buns if they're unstable. Serve with extra remoulade sauce on the side.

INGREDIENTS

2 avocados

sushi vinegar

150 to 200g/5½ to 7oz smoked salmon, sliced

± 85g/8oz lamb's lettuce (or Cos lettuce or baby spinach)

½ a red onion, sliced into thin rings

capers, to taste

sesame seeds

FOR THE REMOULADE SAUCE

4 tbsp mayonnaise

1 tbsp mustard

½ a (small) red onion, finely chopped

3 tbsp gherkins, finely chopped

2 tbsp Amsterdam (or white) pickled cocktail onions, finely chopped

2 tbsp liquid from the pickled cocktail onions

1 tbsp dill or tarragon

pepper and salt, to taste

1 hard-boiled egg

THE WAGYU WAGYME

Wagyu burger bun & classic burger sauce

INGREDIENTS

2 (Wagyu) burgers

2 slices of Cheddar or processed cheese

2 avocados

sushi vinegar

2 red onion slices (5mm/¼in thick)

2 tomato slices (5mm/¼in thick)

2 gherkin slices

watercress or lamb's lettuce

white sesame seeds

FOR THE BURGER SAUCE

1 small shallot, finely chopped

1 tbsp white wine vinegar

1 tbsp finely chopped gherkins

2 tsp yellow mustard

4 tbsp mayonnaise

½ tsp mustard powder

½ tsp smoked paprika powder

1 tsp garlic powder

1 tsp onion powder

½ tsp ground turmeric (for colour)

pepper and salt, to taste

For the burger sauce, put the finely chopped shallot and the white wine vinegar into a small saucepan and simmer gently, stirring occasionally, until the vinegar has evaporated and the onion is soft. Mix this with the rest of the ingredients, and add pepper and salt to taste. Cover and put into the fridge so all the flavours have a chance to develop.

In the meantime, fry one side of the burgers until brown and crispy; flip the burgers and top with cheese. Now continue to fry the burgers until they're done just the way you like.

Make your avocado buns (see page 139 for instructions). Rub the avocado halves with sushi vinegar to keep them from discolouring. On the bottom halves of the buns (which you've filled with burger sauce), place the burgers, the slices of red onion, tomato, and gherkin, and watercress or lamb's lettuce. Top with the other avocado halves and sprinkle with some sesame seeds. If necessary, you can stabilise your burger by inserting a wooden skewer from the top to the bottom.

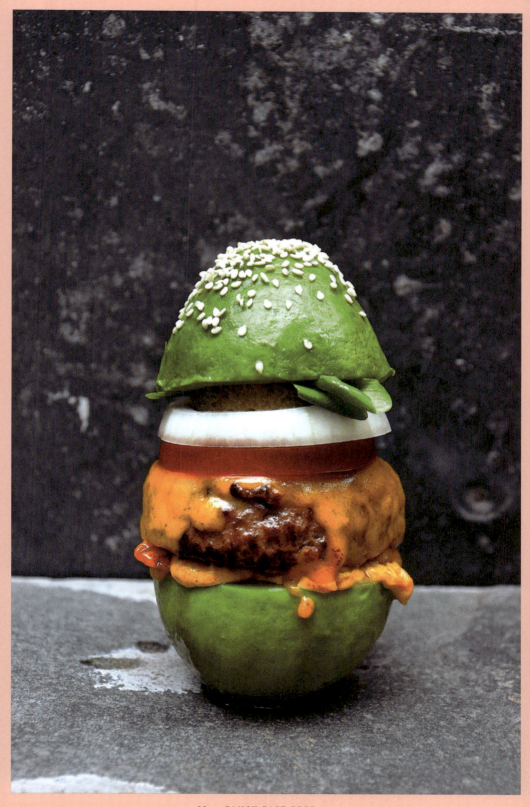

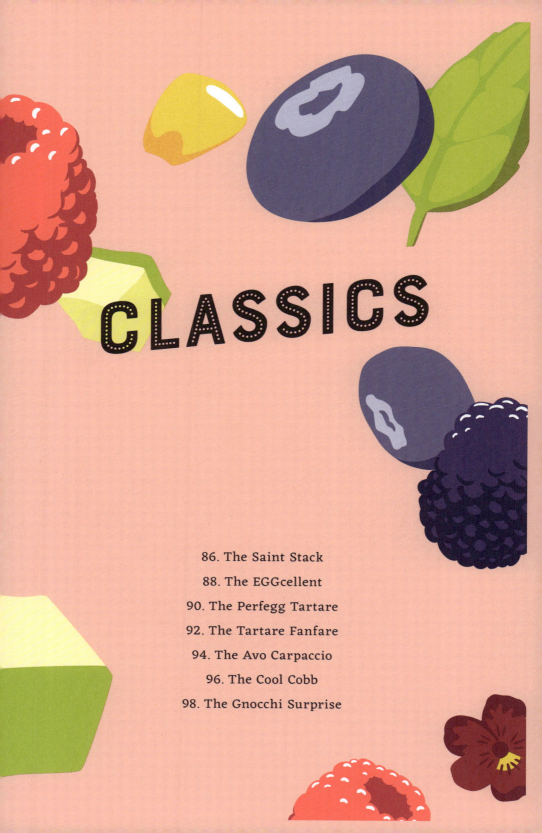

CLASSICS

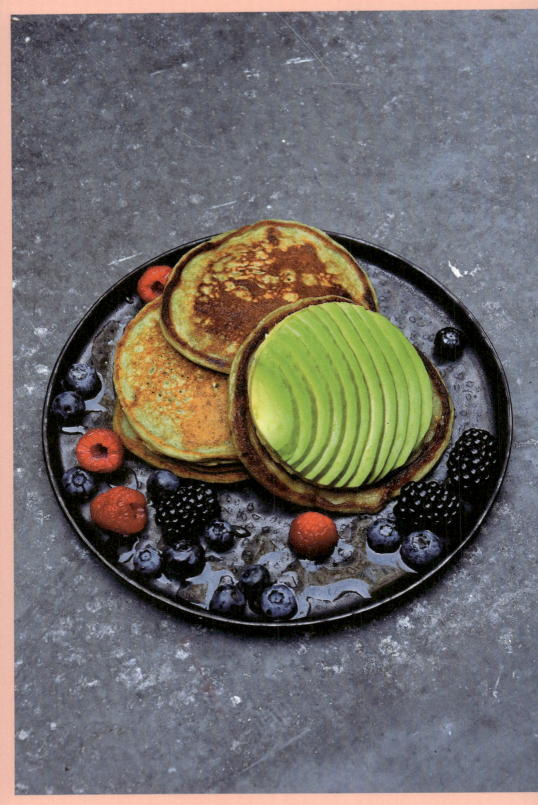

THE SAINT STACK

Stack of vegan matcha pancakes, avocado, berries & maple syrup

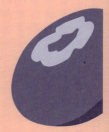
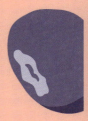

The Sinner Stack and The Saint Stack are two very popular breakfast items at The Avocado Show. Here's the basic recipe for these smash hits. Add the various toppings to turn them into The Sinner or The Saint.

Stir together all the batter ingredients until well mixed.

Heat a little soybean oil in a non-stick frying pan, and fry the pancakes in batches. For nice round pancakes, use a round cutter as a form.

In the meantime, make the round avocado fans. Cut the avocado in half lengthwise, and remove the pit and the peel. Cut thin slices down the length of one of the avocado halves, then press down on this gently to create a kind of fan. Use a cutter to make it nice and round. Repeat with the other avocado half.

On two separate plates, arrange the pancakes attractively into stacks. Use a spatula to place the avocado fans on top of the pancakes. Serve the pancakes with your choice of toppings, and drizzle with a little more maple syrup.

TIP

ARE YOU USING A CUTTER AS A FORM TO MAKE YOUR PANCAKES NICE AND ROUND? MAKE SURE TO GREASE IT WELL BEFORE YOU START

INGREDIENTS

1 avocado

maple syrup, to serve

TOPPINGS SINNER STACK

crispy fried bacon and banana slices

TOPPINGS SAINT STACK

a mixture of berries and the avocado mousse on page 122

FOR THE BATTER

150g/5½oz/heaped 1 cup flour

250ml/9fl oz/1 cup soy milk

2 tbsp maple syrup

½ tbsp soybean oil (+ extra for frying)

2 tsp baking powder

pinch of salt

1 tsp matcha powder

OPTIONAL

a couple of drops of green food colouring

THE EGGCELLENT

Egg, avocado & perfect 60-second hollandaise

Maybe you've never had the courage to make your own hollandaise sauce before. Although it's incredibly delicious, there's a reason this sauce makes people nervous. With this trick it's a breeze, and you'll be done in 60 seconds flat.

P.S. On page 24, there's also a recipe for perfect 60-second truffle mayonnaise.

Poach or soft-boil (6 minutes) the eggs.

Cut the avocados in half lengthwise and remove the pit and the peel. Cut a small piece off the bottom of the avocado halves so they will be more stable once they're on a plate. Rub the halves with a little sushi vinegar. Place two avocado halves on each plate.

Place the egg yolk at the bottom of the jug that came with your hand blender; add the lemon juice, cayenne pepper, and pepper and salt to taste. Melt the butter in a saucepan with a pouring spout, if you have one. Otherwise, pour the melted butter into a small pitcher. Place the hand blender on top of the egg yolk, switch it on, and slowly pour in the hot butter. Carefully raise the hand blender while moving it up and down. A lovely, rich hollandaise sauce will emerge before your very eyes. Have a taste, and add a little more pepper, salt, and/or lemon if you like.

Place the poached or peeled boiled eggs on top of the four avocado halves, and pour about a tablespoon of the hollandaise sauce over each of the eggs. Sprinkle the eggs with pepper and coarse salt to taste. Arrange lamb's lettuce around the avocados, and also decorate with edible flowers and/or Daikon cress if desired. Serve with toast.

UPGRADE

TRY SERVING THIS WITH SMOKED SALMON OR CRISPY BACON!

INGREDIENTS

4 eggs

2 avocados

sushi vinegar

pepper and coarse salt, to taste

lamb's lettuce (or Cos lettuce or baby spinach)

toast, to serve

OPTIONAL

edible flowers and/or daikon cress

FOR THE HOLLANDAISE SAUCE

1 egg yolk, at room temperature

1 tbsp lemon juice (or more, to taste)

a pinch of cayenne pepper

pepper and salt, to taste

100g/3½oz/7 tbsp butter

you will need: a hand blender

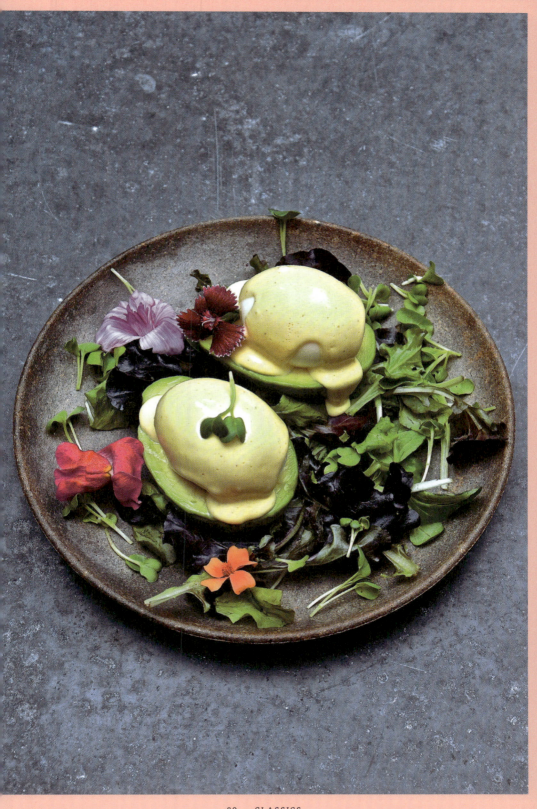

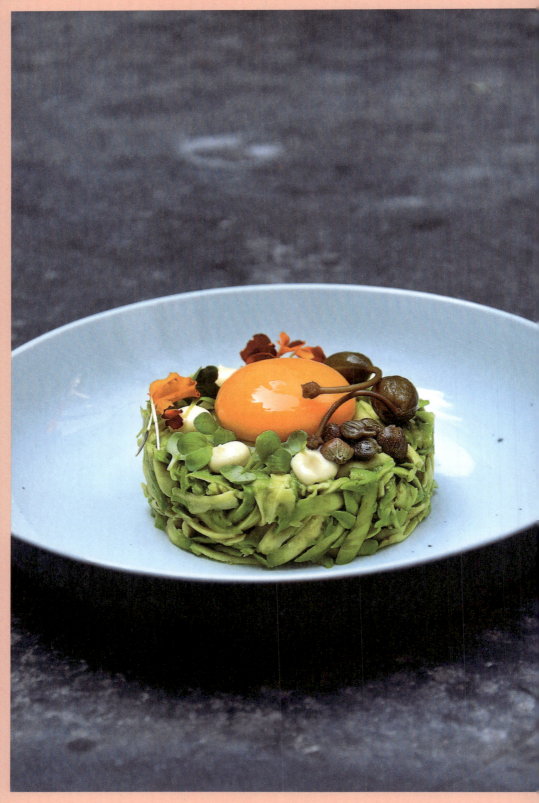

THE PERFEGG TARTARE

Avocado tartare with 65-degree eggs
& anchovy mayo

Tartare is an eternal classic. But this avocado version of tartare gives the dish an entirely new twist.

Preheat the oven to 100°C/200°F/gas ¼. Turn the oven down to 65°C/150°F/gas ¼, place the eggs (still in their shells!) in a small baking dish and put them in the oven. Bake them for 45 minutes.

For the anchovy mayonnaise, puree the mayonnaise, cream cheese and anchovies with a hand blender. Put the mayonnaise into a portioning bottle, piping bag or an empty squeeze bottle (like the ones yellow mustard comes in) so you can pipe on some decorative dots of mayo at the end.

Cut the avocados in half lengthwise, and remove the pit and the peel. Grate the avocados using the coarse side of your grater, and season with the mustard, Worcestershire sauce, sushi vinegar, pepper, and salt.

Serve the avocado as you would tartare. Place a deep cutter in the middle of a plate and spoon in a quarter of the avocado tartare. Press down gently. Repeat for the other three plates.

Carefully peel the eggs – you'll notice that while the egg white is still very soft, the egg yolk is perfect. Remove as much of the egg white as you can, and place the yolk on top of the avocado tartare. Garnish with dabs of anchovy mayonnaise, cress, capers, cornichons, and/or edible flowers.

— SIDES —

SERVE WITH FRESHLY BAKED CRUSTY BREAD, CRACKERS, OR SALTED POPCORN!

INGREDIENTS

4 eggs

4 avocados

1 tsp mustard

a few drops of Worcestershire sauce

1 tbsp sushi vinegar

pepper and salt, to taste

TOPPINGS

cress, capers, cornichons, and/or edible flowerss

you will need: the coarse side of a standing (or box) grater

FOR THE ANCHOVY MAYONNAISE

5 tbsp Japanese Kewpie mayonnaise

2 tbsp cream cheese

1 can (46g/1½oz) anchovies (including the oil)

you will need: a hand blender

THE TARTARE FANFARE

Avocado tartare with mango 'egg yolk' & piccalilli

This vegan version of avocado tartare can be made in a flash. Because you use piccalilli – which contains all of the flavours of steak tartare, from mustard seed to onion – you only need a few ingredients. Instead of an actual egg, here you use an 'egg yolk' made from mango. But it's also delicious with the 65-degree egg from page 90.

Cut the avocados in half lengthwise, and remove the pit and the peel. Grate the avocados using the coarse side of your grater, and season with the sushi vinegar, piccalilli and ginger. Add pepper and salt to taste.

For the egg yolks, slice two thick pieces off the mango. Use a small cutter to cut two 'yolks' out of each mango slice. Don't have the right size cutter? A small glass (about 4cm/1½in in diameter) also works.

Serve the avocado as you would tartare. Place a deep cutter in the middle of a plate and spoon in a quarter of the avocado tartare. Press down gently. Repeat for the other three plates. Place a mango egg yolk in the middle of each tartare, and garnish with edible flowers, cress, finely chopped fresh herbs, and poppyseeds.

— SIDES —

SERVE WITH FRESH CRUSTY BREAD OR CRACKERS

INGREDIENTS

4 avocados

1 tbsp sushi vinegar

4 tbsp piccalilli (+ extra)

fresh ginger (a piece the size of your thumb), finely grated

pepper and salt, to taste

1 mango

TOPPINGS

edible flowers, cress, finely chopped fresh herbs, and poppyseeds

you will need: the coarse side of a standing (or box) grater

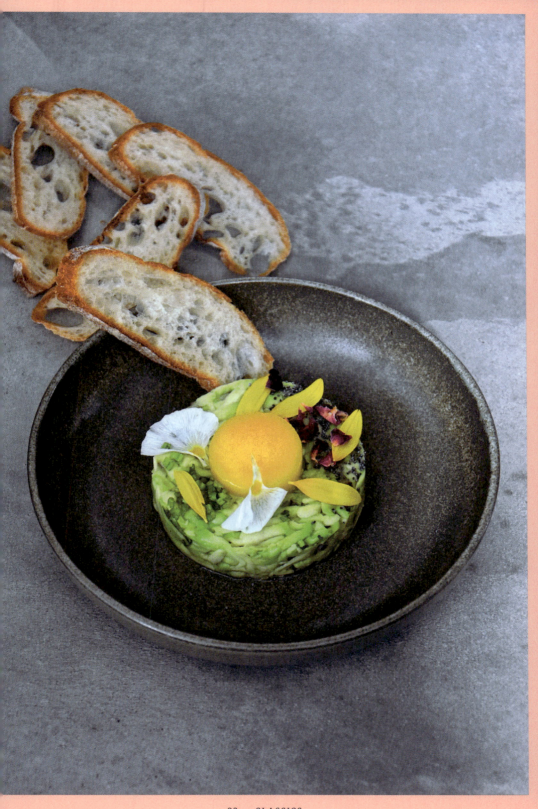

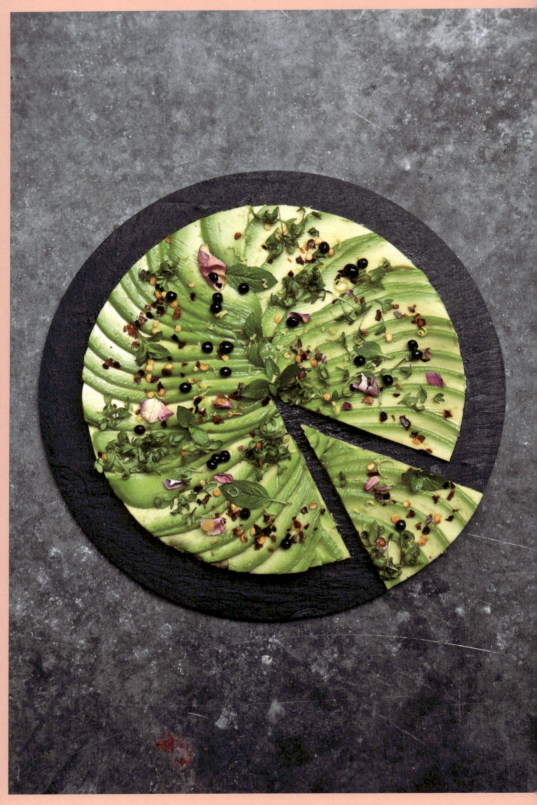

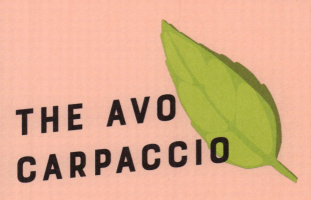

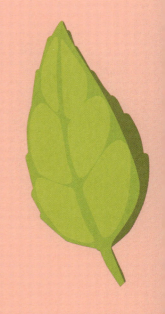

THE AVO CARPACCIO

Carpaccio-style avocado

Carpaccio is traditionally made from thin slices of raw sirloin, served with lemon, olive oil and white truffle or Parmesan cheese. This dish, which you can prepare entirely according to your own tastes, is made from thinly sliced avocado, so it's also suitable for vegans. Avocado has plenty of flavour on its own and a rich, smooth texture so it doesn't necessarily need lots of extras. That's why I'm giving you a basic recipe for this carpaccio, but you can vary the toppings in whatever way you like. The possibilities are endless.

Cut the avocado in half lengthwise, and remove the pit and the peel. Rub the avocado halves with sushi vinegar – this adds a touch of extra flavour and keeps them from discolouring. You can also use lime juice for this purpose.

Place both avocado halves on your cutting board with the rounded side up, and cut them lengthwise into very thin slices. Place both halves on the plate you'll use to serve the dish on. Gently press down on both of the halves and spread them into fans. Place the fans alongside each other, and make the whole thing as round as possible (about 20cm/8in in diameter). Now, find a pan lid that's just a little bit smaller. Place the lid on top of the avocado, and trim off the edges so the avocado circle is completely round. You can use the trimmings to patch your circle here and there. Brush your circle generously with (truffle) olive oil, season with pepper and salt, and garnish with the toppings of your choice.

A nice way to serve the carpaccio is to cut it into wedges as pictured.

INGREDIENTS

1 avocado
sushi vinegar
1 tsp (truffle) olive oil
pepper and salt, to taste

TOPPINGS (FOR INSPIRATION)

balsamic pearls, Parmesan cheese, feta, goat's cheese, grated lime zest, grated lemon zest, chilli flakes, cress, the small leaves from a basil plant, pesto, dried rose petals, edible flowers, balsamic syrup, truffle tapenade, dried ham, smoked fish

you will need: a pan lid and a small brush

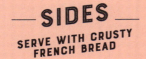

— SIDES —
SERVE WITH CRUSTY FRENCH BREAD

THE COOL COBB

Lots of greens in the mix, with chicken, Cheddar cheese, eggs, crispy bacon, corn & vinaigrette

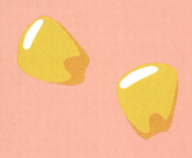

A real American classic. I lived in Canada for two years, where this salad is a firm favourite. Personally, I prefer Cheddar over blue cheese here, but both are a fantastic match for avocado.

In an attractive bowl, mix all of the salad ingredients, except for the avocado. (You could use a vintage baking dish, just like in the photo.)

Mix the ingredients for the vinaigrette and add pepper and salt to taste. Pour the vinaigrette into a small bowl, and tuck this into the salad.

Cut the avocado in half lengthwise, and remove the pit and the peel. Cut one of the halves into thick slices. A nice touch is to use the other half as an extra (edible) sauce bowl. Add the avocado to the salad, and serve.

— SIDES —
THIS MAKES A LOT OF DRESSING, BUT YOU CAN NEVER HAVE TOO MUCH

INGREDIENTS

200g/7oz smoked chicken breast, cubed

2 hard-boiled eggs, peeled and cut in half

100g/3½oz bacon, fried until crisp

100g/3½oz Cheddar cheese (or blue cheese, if you prefer), in small cubes

1 head of lettuce

chives, finely chopped

1 handful of cherry vine tomatoes, cut in half

100g/3½oz corn kernels (from a can)

1 avocado

FOR THE VINAIGRETTE

100ml/3½fl oz/scant ½ cup olive oil

3 tbsp red wine vinegar

1 tbsp Worcestershire sauce

1 tbsp yellow mustard

3 tbsp lemon juice

1 tbsp honey

1 tsp sugar

1 garlic clove, grated

pepper and salt, to taste

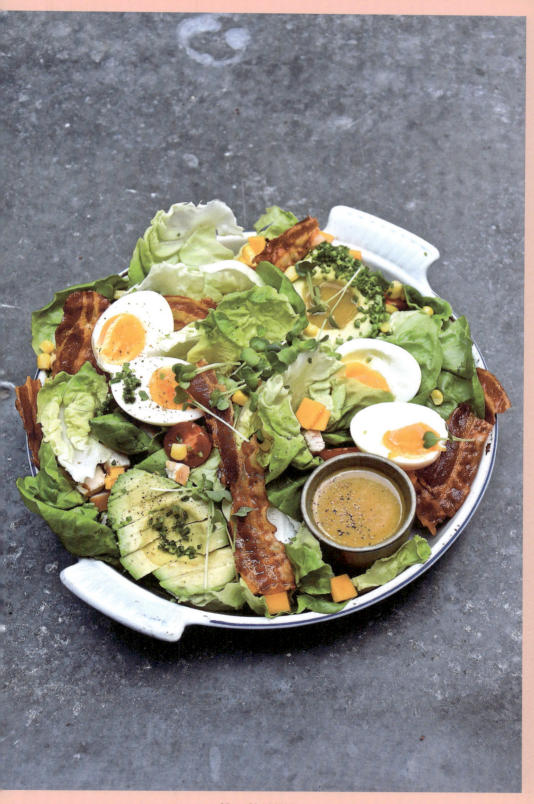

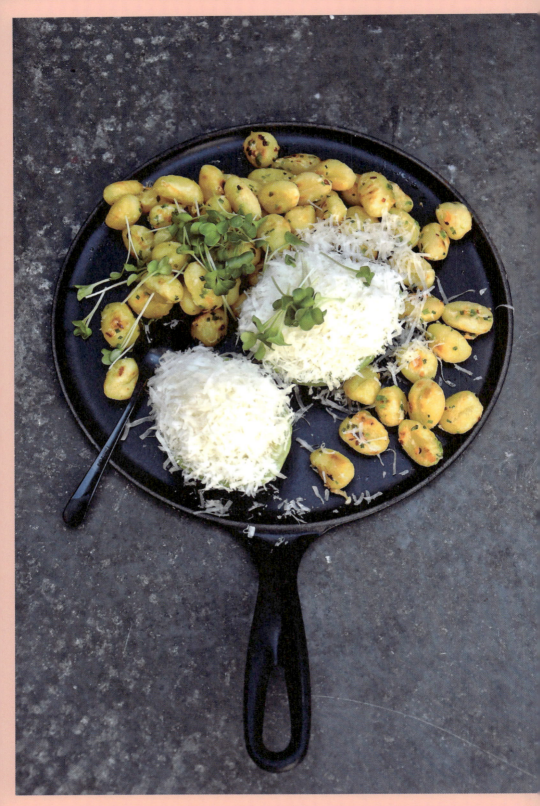

THE GNOCCHI SURPRISE

Crispy gnocchi & avocado truffle bombs

Classic gnocchi are boiled, but if you fry the gnocchi, they become wonderfully crunchy on the outside and tender on the inside: an incredible combination. I always have gnocchi on hand (highly recommended) so I can get a delicious meal on the table in no time. The creamy, nutty flavour of avocado pairs beautifully with the crunchy gnocchi and saltiness of the cheese.

In a non-stick pan, fry the gnocchi in the olive oil over a medium heat, until golden brown and crunchy. This will take about 15 minutes.

In the meantime, make the truffle bombs. To do this, cut the avocado in half lengthwise, and remove the pit and the peel. Cut a small piece off the bottom of both avocado halves, so the bombs will be stable once they're on a plate. Rub the avocado halves with sushi vinegar. Fill the hollows left by the pit with truffle mayonnaise, about 1 tablespoon per half (the amount depends on the size of the pit). Save some truffle mayonnaise to serve on the side.

When the gnocchi are done, add in the grated garlic, chilli flakes, parsley or chives, and half of the Parmesan cheese, and fry for another minute.

Place the avocado halves onto the platter or onto the plates you'll use to serve the dish. Distribute the other half of the Parmesan cheese over both avocado halves, and top with a little cress. Now add the hot gnocchi to the platter or plates, and drizzle with a little olive oil. Serve with truffle mayonnaise on the side.

Instead of using a platter or plates, I sometimes use one of my nicest baking dishes or pans for serving. Pictured here is a cast-iron crêpe pan.

SIDES

THE TRUFFLE BOMB IS ALSO DELICIOUS WITH A SALAD, OR AS A DIP SERVED WITH CRUDITÉS

INGREDIENTS

1 packet (500g/1lb 2oz) gnocchi

2 tbsp olive oil, for frying (+ extra for serving)

1 avocado

sushi vinegar

± 2 tbsp truffle mayonnaise (+ extra for serving), your favourite shop-bought kind or homemade (see page 24)

1 small garlic clove, grated

1 tsp chilli flakes

a few sprigs of fresh parsley or chives, finely chopped

50g/1¾oz Parmesan cheese, finely grated

cress

OPTIONAL

Parma ham (add in at the very end, while frying)

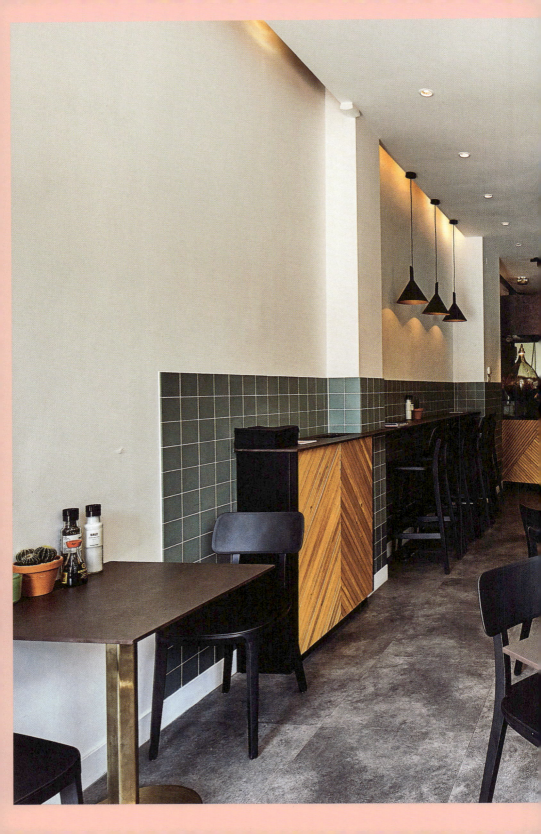

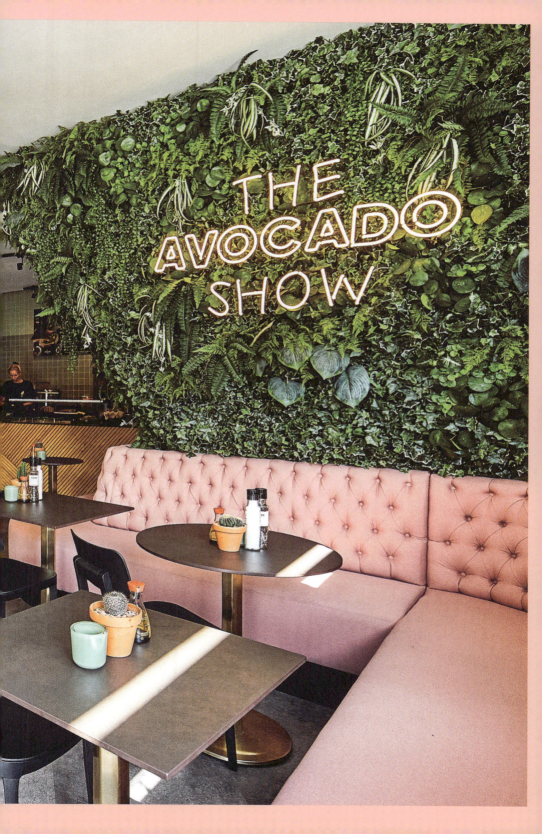

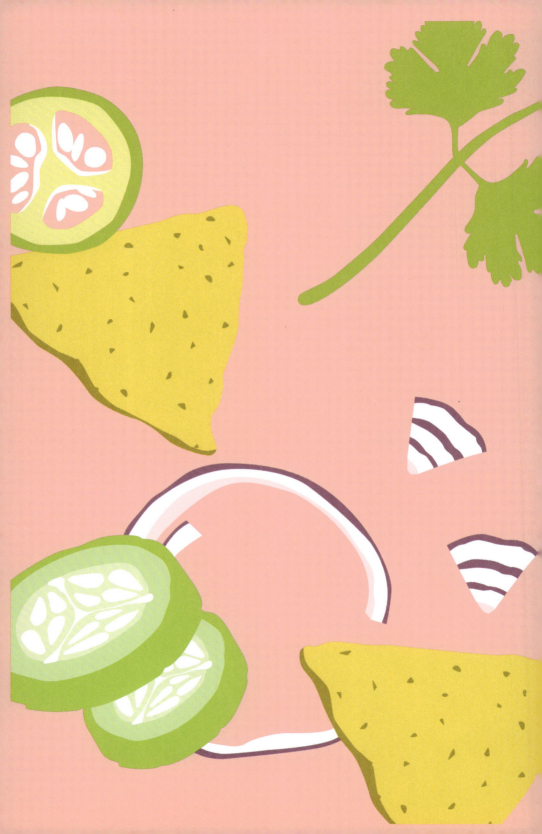

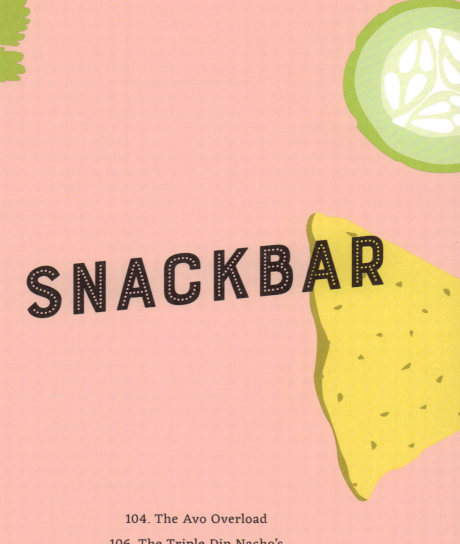

SNACKBAR

THE AVO OVERLOAD

Avocado bites with berbere

Berbere is an Ethiopian spice mixture, hot and fiery and full of flavour. I always keep my homemade blend on hand, and often use it in combination with avocado. As you can see in the picture, I use berbere in a simple way here, as the only topping for the avocado. But it's also very delicious and pretty sprinkled on plain mashed avocado on toast!

HOW TO MAKE THE BERBERE

For the berbere, toast the chilli flakes, coriander seeds, allspice berry, clove, black peppercorns and cumin seed in a dry frying pan. Allow to cool briefly. Grind this in a pestle and mortar or spice grinder with the rest of the ingredients until everything is well ground and blended. Taste, and add more salt if necessary.

PUTTING TOGETHER THE SNACK BOARD

The fuller your board, the more attractive it will be, so don't use a board that's too big. Make avocado roses (see page 136), scoop out small avocado balls with a melon baller, make a pixelated avocado (see page 140), and also cut some avocado wedges if you like. Various shapes and textures are a feast for the eye, and if things overlap, it only adds to the appeal. Sprinkle a little berbere over all of the avocado bites, and add a small dish of extra berbere to the board.

Room for a few more snacks? Add a couple of bowls with some of the other dips from this book. Is your board still not full? Tuck in some fresh herbs, olives, a little rocket (arugula) and maybe a bunch of radishes (always a nice touch, and they taste good too). Different kinds of crackers and a selection of cold meats and cheeses provide the ultimate finishing touch.

INGREDIENTS

avocados (pictured here are 4 avocados)

FOR THE BERBERE

1 tsp chilli flakes

1 tsp coriander seeds

1 allspice berry

1 clove

2 black peppercorns

¼ tsp cumin seed

1 tsp smoked sweet paprika powder

2 tsp mild paprika powder

1 tsp ground ginger

½ tsp ground cinnamon

½ tsp garlic powder

pinch of cardamom

¼ tsp fenugreek

1 tsp onion powder

1 tsp sea salt

½ tsp ground turmeric

OPTIONAL

breadsticks, to serve on the side

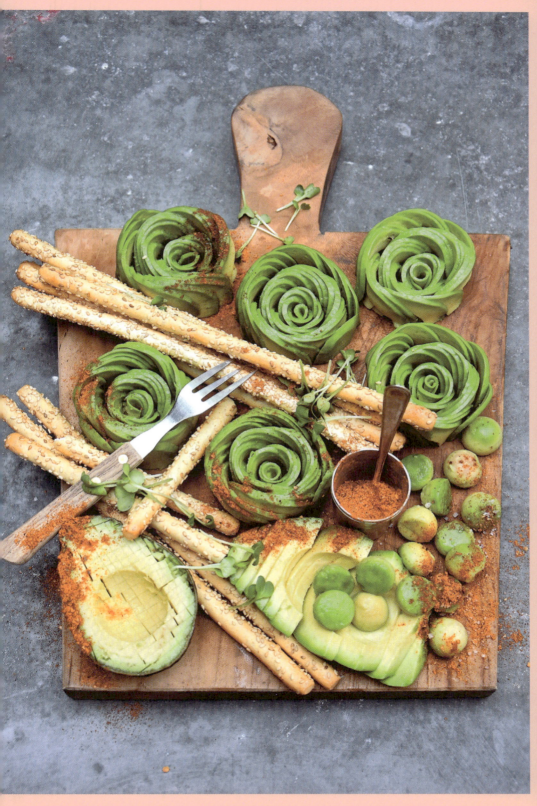

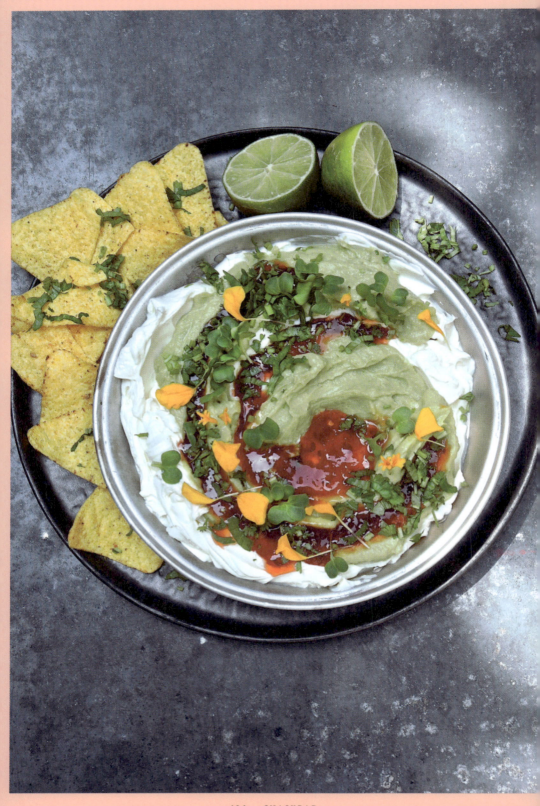

THE TRIPLE DIP NACHO'S

Nachos, cream cheese, avocado spread & hot chilli sauce

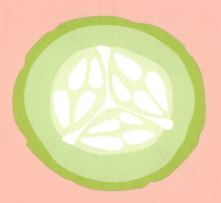

For years, this snack has been making encore appearances at drinks parties, celebrations and other gatherings. What's more, people at my house count on me to make it (amongst other avocado dishes). It's always a hit, and couldn't be easier. By the way, it's also good without coriander (cilantro), seeing that not everyone is crazy about it. This is why I often put coriander on only half of the dip, and leave it off of the other half.

Mash or puree the avocados along with the lime juice and a little salt to make a smooth spread.

Spread the cream cheese onto a plate with a rim, or spoon it into a dish. Spread the avocado mixture over this, but don't cover it completely – it's nice if the white of the cream cheese is still visible. Finish with a generous splash of chilli sauce in the middle. Sprinkle with the finely chopped coriander, daikon cress and flower petals. Serve with the tortilla chips.

Before you cut your lime, press it down onto the worktop with your hand, and roll it back and forth a few times. This will make it easier to juice.

INGREDIENTS

2 avocados

juice of 1 lime

salt

± 200g/7oz/scant 1 cup cream cheese

± 100ml/3½fl oz/scant ½ cup chilli sauce

1 small bunch of coriander (cilantro), leaves and stems finely chopped

daikon cress

edible flower petals

1 bag (of around 200g/7oz) tortilla chips, to serve

THE SO EXTRA AVO SPREAD

Loaded avocado spread with watermelon, feta, olives, edible flowers & cress

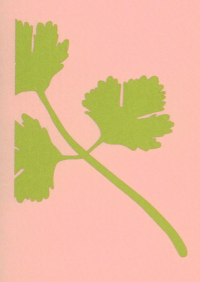

INGREDIENTS

2 avocados

grated zest of ½ small unsprayed lemon

juice of 1 small unsprayed lemon

1 tbsp sushi vinegar

1 small garlic clove, grated

1 or 2 tbsp tahini, to taste

salt, to taste

TOPPINGS

100g/3½oz white cheese (feta), crumbled

a handful of olives

1 small bunch of coriander (cilantro), leaves and stems finely chopped

½ a small watermelon, cut into small cubes

¼ red onion, finely chopped

cress

you will need: a food processor

A quick and cheerful dip to serve with drinks or at a BBQ. The recipe for this spread is based on hummus, but I use avocado instead of chickpeas. The basic ingredients for hummus make for a beautiful combination, even without the chickpeas.

In a food processor, blend together all the ingredients for the avocado spread. Taste, and add salt if necessary. Spread the avocado mixture on an attractive plate, and garnish with the toppings.

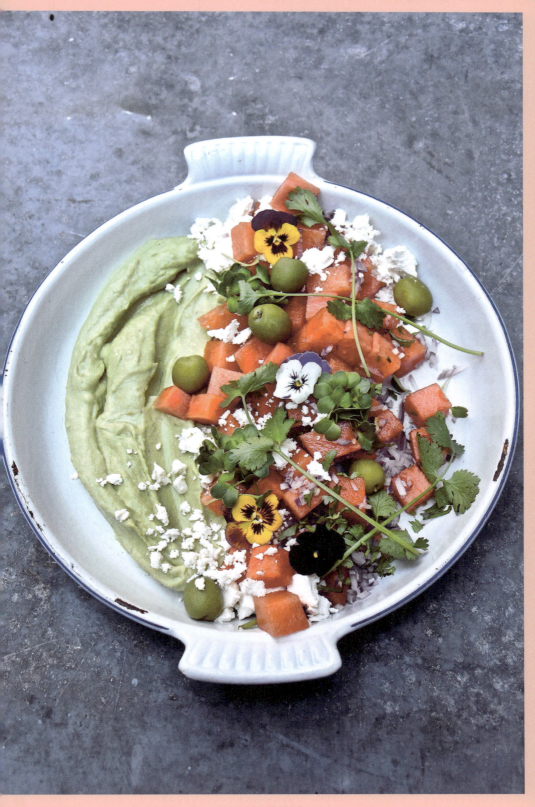

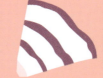

THE AVOCADO SHOW CLASSIC

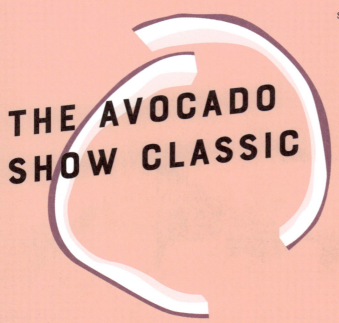

Cut the avocados in half lengthwise, and remove the pit and the peel.

In a bowl, mash the flesh of the avocado together with all the other ingredients, making it as chunky or as smooth as you like. Taste, and season with pepper and salt. Serve on toast, decorated with edible flowers and cress, or with tortilla chips.

— TIP —
GUACAMOLE HAS TO BE CHUNKY, NOT SMOOTH

INGREDIENTS

2 avocados

½ a red onion, finely chopped

½ a red chilli pepper, finely chopped

1 small bunch of fresh coriander (cilantro), leaves and stems finely chopped

1 small sweet red (bell) pepper, cut into (5mm/¼in) squares

juice of 2 limes

grated zest of 1 unsprayed lime

pepper and salt, to taste

OPTIONAL

toast, edible flowers and cress, or tortilla chips, to serve

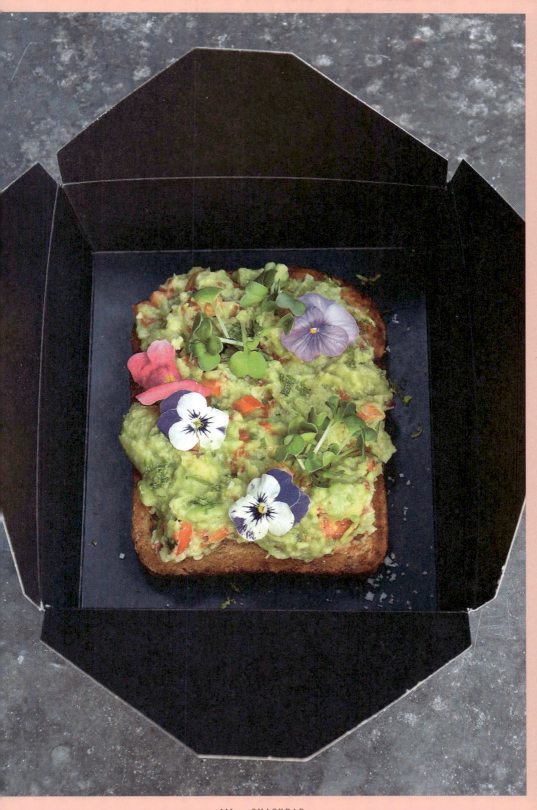

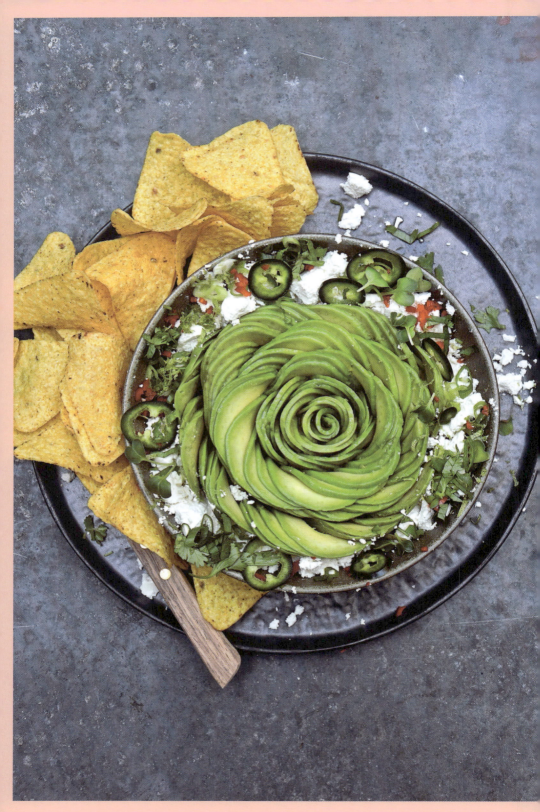

THE FOODDECO SPICY FETA

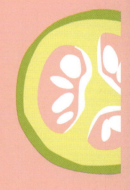

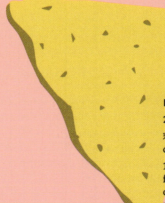

Make an XXL avocado rose from the two avocados. See page 136 for how to make an avocado rose, with one exception: in step 3, line up the four rows of avocado to make one long row. Continue with the remaining steps.

Place the avocado rose on a large, attractive plate. Arrange all the other ingredients around the rose. Serve with tortilla chips and your nicest fork. Have one of your guests finish the guacamole by mashing all the ingredients together. Add a little more pepper and salt to taste.

So convenient: if your avocados are nice and ripe, all you have to do is slice them in half and remove the pit – then just give them a squeeze and the flesh pops right out.

INGREDIENTS

2 avocados

½ a red chilli pepper, finely chopped

1 jalapeño pepper, one half finely chopped and the other half sliced into thin rings

1 small garlic clove, grated

1 spring onion (scallion), finely chopped

juice and zest of 1 unsprayed lime

100g/3½oz white cheese/feta

1 small bunch of coriander (cilantro), leaves and stems finely chopped

pepper and salt, to taste

tortilla chips, to serve

THE HOLY TRUFFLE GUACAMOLY

You have to play around with the flavours and ingredients a bit here, so it doesn't end up being too salty or too acidic and yet has enough truffle flavour. Every truffle tapenade and truffle oil tastes different, so add a little more or a little less to taste. It also depends on how you're planning to serve this guacamole. As part of a sandwich (say, with bacon), the guacamole needs a little more truffle. The quantities below are perfect for a guacamole that will be served as a dip.

Cut the avocados in half lengthwise, and remove the pit. Squeeze or spoon out the flesh of both avocados into a bowl. Mix the other ingredients into the avocado. Taste, and season with pepper and salt.

— TIP —
USE A POTATO MASHER TO MASH THE AVOCADOS

INGREDIENTS

2 avocados

1 tbsp truffle tapenade (or more, to taste)

1 tbsp truffle oil (or more, to taste)

1 tbsp lemon juice

1 spring onion (scallion), finely chopped

½ a garlic clove, grated

pepper and (truffle) salt, to taste

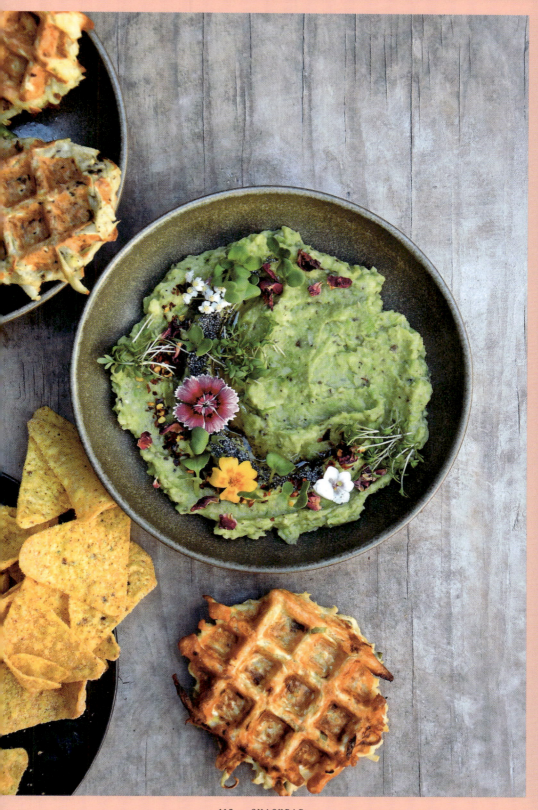

AVOCADO
GLUTEN F
DAIRY FRE
VEGETARIA
CHOLESTE
BASICALLY

ARE
REE,
E, VEGAN,
N AND
ROL-FREE.
PERFECT.

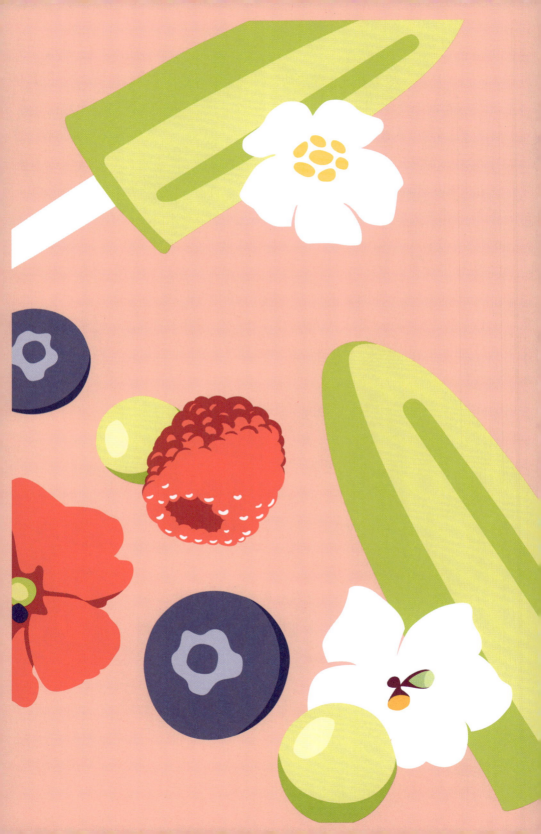

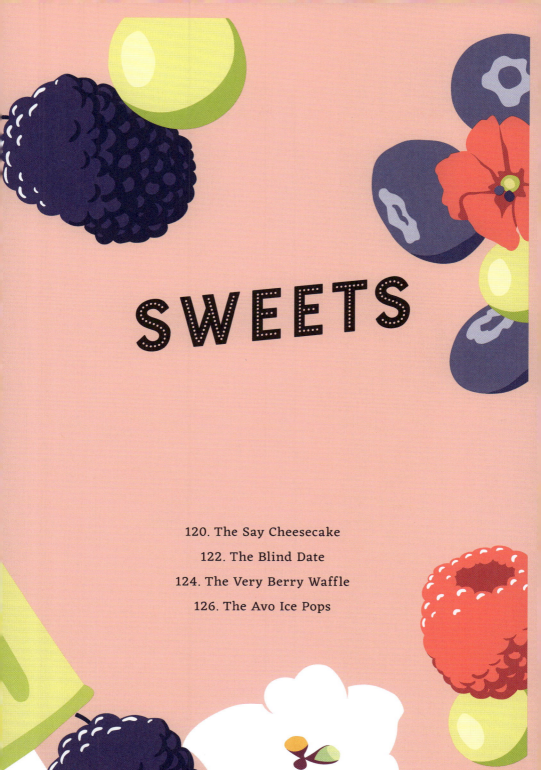

SWEETS

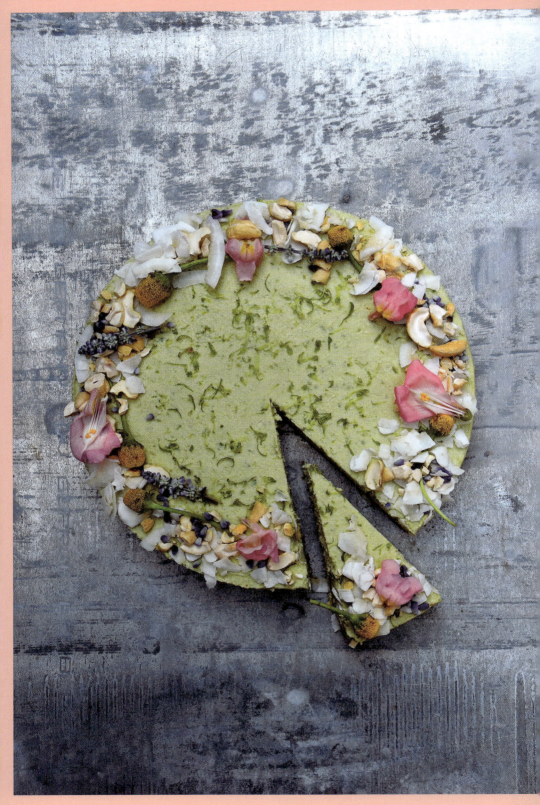

THE SAY CHEESECAKE

Avocado & lime cheesecake

For children's birthdays, I decorate this cake with plastic giraffes, parrots, flamingos and Duplo bricks. It's always a hit. But on 'just-because-you-feel-like-having-cheesecake' days, you can decorate this photogenic cake with flowers, grated coconut and grated lime zest – just like in the picture.

Soak the cashews in water in a covered dish; leave overnight in the fridge. Before you start making the crust, transfer them to a strainer and drain well.

To make the crust, coarsely grind the almonds in a food processor. Add the other crust ingredients, and blitz until well blended. Distribute this mixture over the bottom of the cake pan (you don't need to grease the pan), and press down firmly.

Wash the food processor, and grind the cashews into a butter, then add the rest of the ingredients for the filling and mix until completely smooth. Pour the filling onto the crust, cover the cheesecake, and put it in the fridge to set for at least 4 hours.

Remove the cake from the cake pan, and decorate with your choice of toppings.

INGREDIENTS

FOR THE CRUST

175g/6oz/1⅓ cups blanched almonds

200g/7oz pitted dates

75g/2½oz/1 cup grated coconut (+ extra for decorating)

FOR THE FILLING

200g/7oz/1⅔ cups cashews

flesh of 2 avocados

150ml/5fl oz/scant ⅔ cup coconut cream (from a can or carton)

125g/4½oz coconut oil, melted

juice and grated zest of 4 unsprayed limes (save a little grated zest for decorating)

3 tbsp maple syrup (or honey, but then the cake will no longer be vegan)

TOPPINGS

edible flowers, grated lime zest, grated coconut, and/or finely chopped cashews (as desired)

you will need: a food processor and a spring-form cake pan (± 22cm/8½in in diameter)

THE BLIND DATE

Avocado mousse with citrus & vanilla with a nut-anise seed crunch, served as an avocado

Did you know that the flesh directly beneath the skin is the healthiest part of the avocado? Make sure you use a spoon to scrape it all out. Although this recipe calls for four avocados, you'll only need the shells from two of them, which you'll use to serve the mousse. There are lots of ways to use the surplus avocado flesh – for example, it's ideal for making one of the guacamoles (see pages 110–115).

Preheat the oven to 160°C/315°F/gas 2–3.

Cut the avocados in half lengthwise, remove the pits, and scoop the flesh out of the shells. You'll be using the shells later as serving dishes, so make sure to keep them whole.

Blend all the filling ingredients (remember: use the flesh of only two of the avocados) in the food processor until smooth. Put the filling in the fridge for at least 30 minutes to set.

In the meantime, start making the date crumble. Mix together the flaked almonds, sesame seeds and anise seed. Spread the mixture on baking parchment and bake this in the oven for about 15 minutes until golden brown and crunchy, while stirring it every 5 minutes. This mixture smells wonderful!

Remove the almond mixture from the oven and allow to cool, then grind it together with the dates in the food processor to make a coarse crumble. From this mixture, form four balls the size of an avocado pit, and set the rest aside. You will need approximately 3 tablespoons of the crumble mixture for every pit.

Spoon the mousse into the eight avocado shells. Make sure the tops are completely smooth, so that they look just like avocado halves. On four of the halves, place a ball on the spot where the pit would be, and sprinkle a little of the reserved crumble over the other four halves. Each serving should include a half with a pit and a half with the crumble. Garnish with edible flowers if you like.

Congratulations if you manage to have some filling left over to serve to your guests – it's very tempting to keep eating it straight from the food processor.

FOR THE FILLING

4 avocados (from 2 of the avocados, you'll only need the shells)

grated zest of 1 unsprayed orange

juice and grated zest of 1 unsprayed lemon

100ml/3½fl oz/scant ½ cup agave syrup

1 tbsp maple syrup

100g/3½oz coconut oil, melted

2 tsp vanilla extract

FOR THE DATE CRUMBLE

100g/3½oz/1¼ cups flaked almonds

50g/1¾oz/⅓ cup white sesame seeds

2 tsp anise seed

100g/3½oz (around 5) dates, pitted

OPTIONAL

edible flowers, to garnish

you will need: a food processor

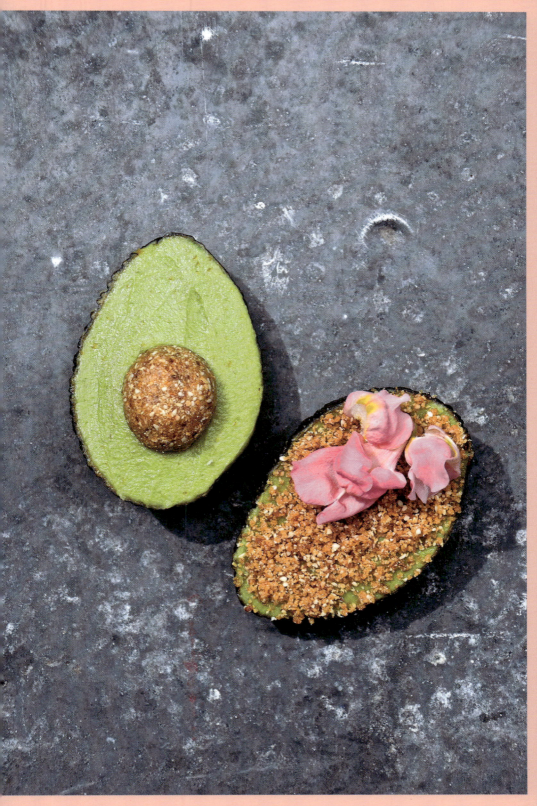

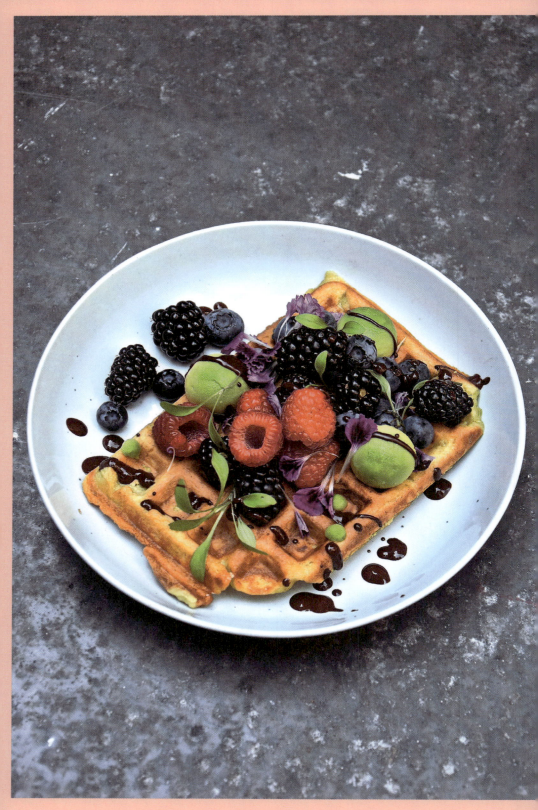

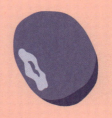

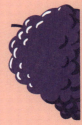

THE VERY BERRY WAFFLE

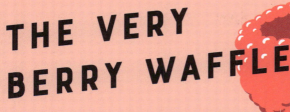

Avocado waffle with berries, avocado, chocolate sauce & cress

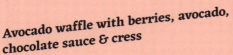

INGREDIENTS
FOR THE WAFFLE BATTER

100g/3½oz/¾ cup flour

100g/3½fl oz/scant ½ cup coconut yoghurt

1 egg

2 or 3 tsp vanilla extract

1 avocado, pureed

1 tsp baking powder

40g/1½oz/⅓ cup icing sugar

pinch of salt

1 tbsp olive oil (+ extra for greasing)

FOR THE CHOCOLATE SAUCE

30g/1oz dark chocolate (70% cocoa solids)

TOPPINGS

berries, avocado berries, edible flowers and Ghoa cress

The 'avocado berries' in the photo are simple to make using a melon baller, and combine nicely with real berries.

Mix together all the batter ingredients – you can use a food processor for this if you like.

Grease the waffle iron with the olive oil and pour the batter in. Bake the waffles until brown and crisp. The baking time will vary based on your waffle iron, as every iron is different. If your iron makes just one waffle at a time, use half the batter for baking the first waffle, and use the other half for baking the second waffle.

Meanwhile, melt the chocolate in a bain-marie. Arrange the berries and the avocado berries on the crisp waffles. Drizzle them with the chocolate sauce. Decorate the waffles with edible flowers and Ghoa cress, if desired.

For a savoury version, leave out the sugar, vanilla extract and chocolate sauce. Substitute smoked salmon or guacamole (made using one of the recipes in this book) for the berries.

you will need: a waffle iron, food processor and a melon baller

THE AVO ICE POPS

Creamy avocado-vanilla ice pops

These creamy ice pops are so easy to make, and there's no ice cream maker involved. You only need five ingredients and a little patience.

Slice the vanilla pod in half lengthwise and use the tip of a knife to scrape out the seeds. Bring the coconut milk, honey, vanilla seeds, and vanilla pod to a boil, and allow to simmer for about 5 minutes. Let the mixture cool (leave in the vanilla pod, so it can release even more flavour). Once it has cooled, remove the vanilla pod from the infused coconut milk.

Cut the avocados in half lengthwise, remove the pit, and squeeze or scoop out the avocado flesh into the food processor. Using a fine grater, grate in the lime zest. Cut the limes in half and add the lime juice as well. Mix the ingredients in the food processor until well blended.

Fill around 12 ice cream moulds with the avocado mixture, and freeze overnight.

— **TIP** —
YOU CAN ALSO USE VANILLA EXTRACT INSTEAD OF A VANILLA POD

INGREDIENTS

1 vanilla pod

500ml/17fl oz/2 cups coconut milk

150g/5½oz/scant ½ cup honey

3 avocados

2 unsprayed limes

you will need: a food processor and ice cream moulds

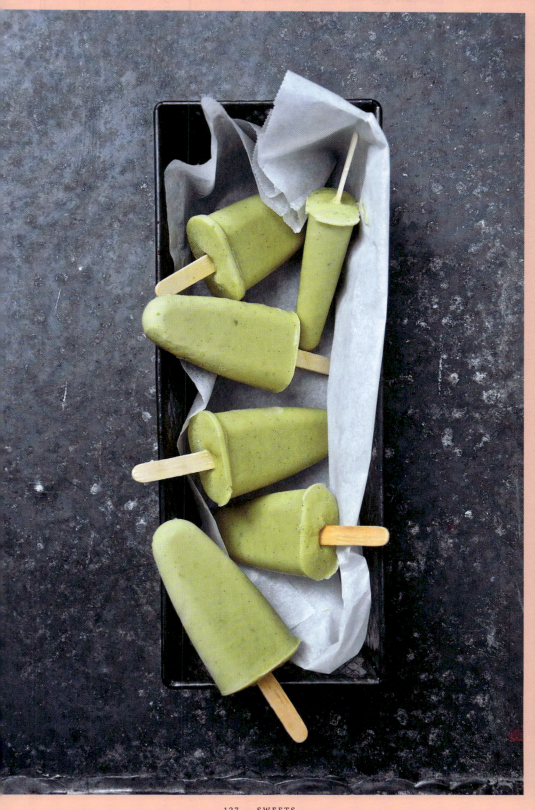

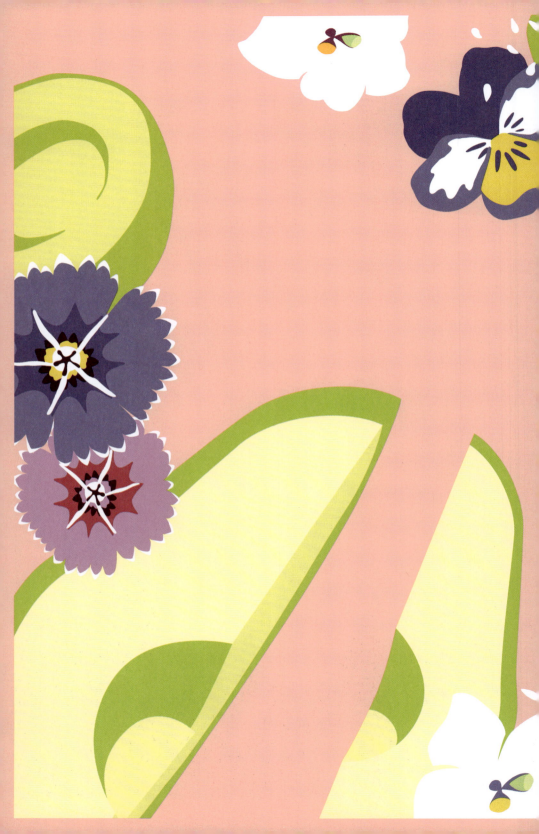

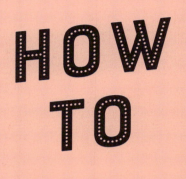

HOW
TO

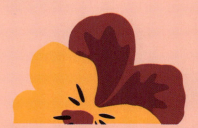

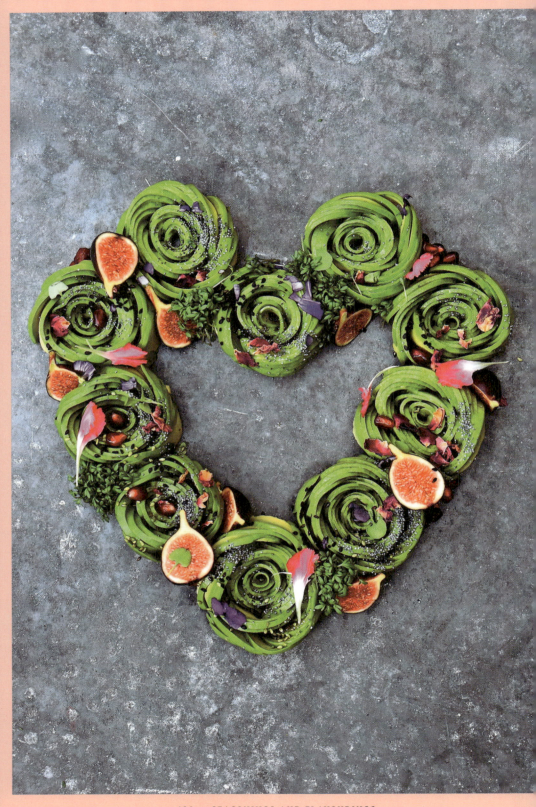

SEASONINGS AND FLAVOURINGS

There are a number of flavours you'll often find in combination with avocado, such as lime, coriander (cilantro) and chilli pepper. But the possibilities are endless. Have you ever tried avocado with tarragon? Or avocado with homemade berbere, an Ethiopian spice mixture? Truffle and avocado are also a match made in heaven, so you'll find a number of dishes that use this lovely combination.

Coffee goes unexpectedly well with avocado. The combination is quite remarkable, so do try drinking a freshly brewed espresso along with your avocado on toast.

The colour of balsamic vinegar (see Balsamico Fantastico on page 58) contrasts beautifully with the green of the avocado. Also, I love the flavour of this extraordinary vinegar with its perfect balance of sweet and sour! Do make sure you buy the good-quality vinegar or syrup from Modena.

Coconut combines very well with avocado, which is why I always have coconut yoghurt, grated coconut, coconut flakes and coconut oil on hand.

There are always frozen bananas in the freezer, ready to use for a delicious milkshake with avocado (see page 72). I highly recommend these milkshakes, especially during the busy morning rush hours with kids.

I always have sushi vinegar on hand, and use it in almost everything I make with avocado. Sushi vinegar is a combination of rice vinegar, sugar and salt. It gives the avocado extra flavour, and also keeps the avocado from turning brown. In the 'How to' chapter, you can read how I rub the avocado halves with sushi vinegar for each of my creations. I also use sushi vinegar as an ingredient in dressings and sauces.

PRESENTATION

In addition to seasonings and flavourings, I love using beautiful ingredients – they give dishes that special touch.

Besides flavour, turmeric also adds a vibrant colour to your dish. And the colour of grated lime zest is very attractive next to the green of the avocado.

I adore all kinds of cress, and one of my favourites is daikon cress. I love it for its flavour, but also for its heart-shaped leaves. I've always got some of it in the fridge. You can use it in any number of dishes, to transform your creation into a real eyecatcher! If you can't get cress, you can also use a basil plant. To add refinement to a dish, pick the smallest leaves of the plant (at the bottom of the stem) and you've got 'basil cress'.

Edible flowers come in a wide range of colours, varieties and sizes, each with their own flavour, from violets and pansies to carnations and roses. They can make any dish special. Fresh edible flowers are glorious, of course, but they aren't always available. This is why I'm also a fan of the dried variety – dried rose petals are often easy to find. I keep them in a crystal jar in my kitchen, which is also very decorative.

INGREDIENTS I ALWAYS HAVE ON HAND TO CREATE STUNNING PLATES OF FOOD (AND TO ADD SOME EXTRA FLAVOUR)

sesame seeds (black, white and green)

poppyseeds

dried rose petals (or fresh edible flowers)

cress

grated coconut

chilli flakes

fresh herbs: coriander (cilantro), basil, mint and leaf celery

various spices, including ground cumin, paprika powder, cayenne pepper, ground turmeric and curry powder

sushi vinegar, for that touch of shine and flavour

various seeds & nuts

balsamic syrup and balsamic vinegar

tahini

limes

lemons

fresh peppers: red chilli peppers and jalapeños

pepper and salt, of various kinds and colours

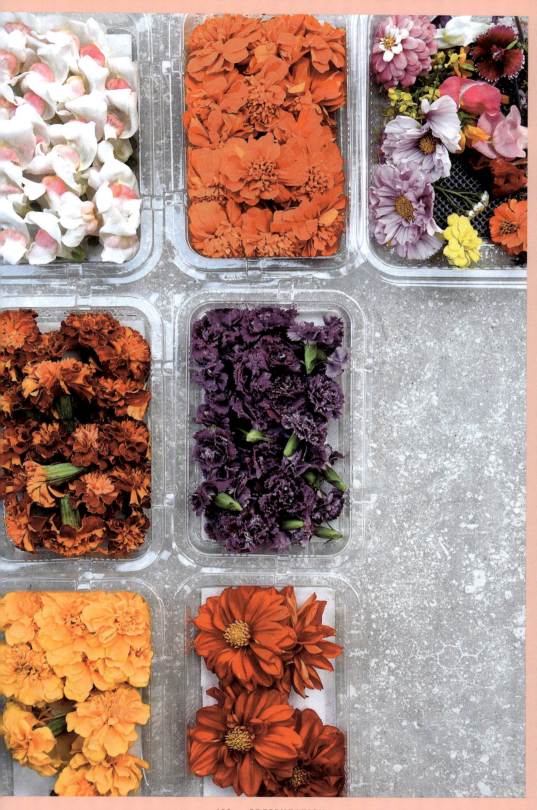

HOW TO...
PEEL AN
AVOCADO

Should you peel with a knife or by hand? By hand, please.

1. Cut the avocado in half lengthwise with a sharp knife and remove the pit. The safest and easiest way to do this is by hand or with a spoon.

2. Now try and find a spot where you can easily get your fingernails between the flesh of the avocado and the peel. Start peeling, and remove the whole thing – just like you would do with a banana.

3. By following these instructions, you'll keep your avocado intact and as smooth as possible. Perfect for making something like an avocado garden or avocado rose. Don't forget to rub the avocado halves with sushi vinegar, before using them to make something from this book.

YOU WILL NEED

avocado

sharp knife

sushi vinegar

—— TIP ——
ARE THERE STILL SOME
UNPEELED BITS OR A FEW
DARK SPOTS? CAREFULLY
REMOVE THEM WITH A
KNIFE OR VEGETABLE
PEELER

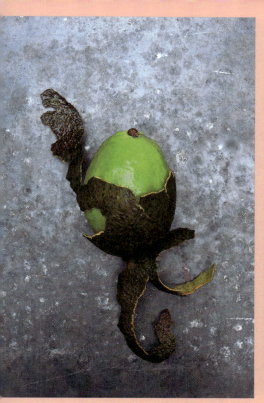

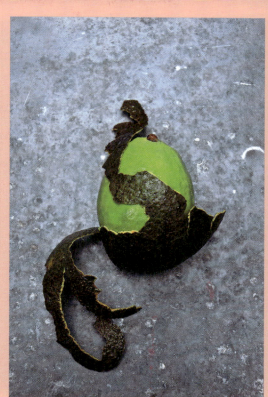

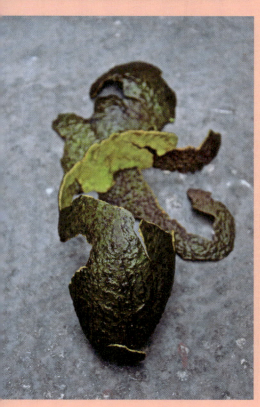

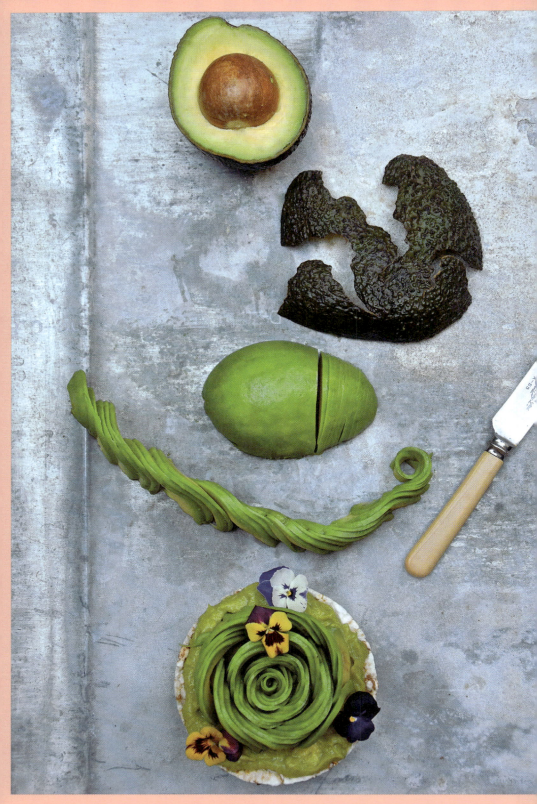

HOW TO...
MAKE AN
AVOCADO ROSE

An avocado rose brightens every plate. So how do you actually make an avocado rose? It only takes four steps! It's easier than you think, and with a little practice, you'll master it in no time.

1. Cut the avocado in half lengthwise, and remove the pit and the peel. See page 134 for tips.

2. Place one half of the avocado (which you've rubbed with sushi vinegar) on your cutting board with the rounded side up. Using a sharp knife, cut the avocado crosswise into very thin slices of around 2mm/⅟₁₆in.

3. Arrange the slices (overlapping them a bit) into a long row, then roll it up to form a rose.

4. Use the spatula to move the avocado rose from your cutting board to its final destination. In this book you'll find lots of different recipes that feature an avocado rose, from toast to guacamole and salads.

Would you like to save the other half of the avocado? Then don't remove the pit, and rub the flesh with sushi vinegar – this prevents it from turning brown.

YOU WILL NEED
cutting board
sharp knife
½ an avocado per rose
sushi vinegar
flat spatula

TOPPINGS
(water)cress, edible flowers, chilli flakes to taste (not pictured)

HOW TO... MAKE AN AVOCADO CROWN

This mostly is just like making an avocado rose, but instead of rolling it up completely, you form it into a large circle.

1. Cut the avocado in half lengthwise, and remove the pit and the peel. Place the avocado halves on your cutting board with the rounded sides up, and remove a small piece from both ends of each half. You can go ahead and eat these now.

2. Place one half of the avocado (which you've rubbed with sushi vinegar) on your cutting board with the rounded side up. Cut the avocado crosswise into very thin slices of around 2mm/1⁄16in.

3. Arrange the slices (overlapping them a bit) into a long row and form this into a circle (of around 12cm/4½in in diameter) to make a crown – or rather, a bowl.

4. Use a spatula to move your crown from the cutting board to a plate, and fill it with the ingredients for the poke bowl. See page 52 for The Vegan Poke Show, and page 50 for The Avo Poke Show with marinated salmon.

In addition to poke bowls, you can use the crown for all sorts of things. Try filling the bowl with scrambled eggs, a fresh salad, or guacamole.

YOU WILL NEED

cutting board

sharp knife

½ an avocado per crown

sushi vinegar

flat spatula

HOW TO...
MAKE AN
AVOCADO BUN

1. Cut the avocado in half widthwise – you're actually circling around the pit with your knife. Twist the two halves apart. You now have the top and the bottom of the 'bun'.

2. Remove the pit, and cut a small piece off the underside of the bottom half so it will be a bit more stable.

3. Peel both avocado halves, and rub them with sushi vinegar. If you find these two halves a little high for a 'bun' when stacked, cut a thick slice from the bottom of both halves. This will also make the bun more stable after assembly.

4. If you spoon some sauce onto the plate and place the bottom half of the burger bun on top of the sauce, your burger bun will stay put without sliding. Fill the hollow left by the pit with the sauce, and start building your burger. For further instructions on how to assemble the burger, see the Wagyu burger bun with hamburger sauce on page 82, the carrot dog on page 78, and the smoked salmon sandwich & remoulade on page 80.

If you like, you can insert a long (wooden) skewer from top to bottom through the burger; but do it carefully to make sure your burger bun remains whole.

Experiment with the different kinds of sesame seeds: use white, black, or green sesame seeds, or a combination of all three..

YOU WILL NEED
cutting board
sharp knife
1 avocado for 1 burger
sushi vinegar

OPTIONAL
(wooden) skewer

HOW TO...
MAKE A PIXELATED
AVOCADO

There are two ways to make a pixelated avocado: the easy way (with the peel) and a somewhat more complicated way (without the peel). The first way is useful if you want to be quick, the second way is more precise. To keep it simple, cut the avocado in half lengthwise, and remove the pit. Cut tiny blocks while still in the peel and easily scoop the pixelated avocado from the peel with a spoon. For the more complicated way:

1. Cut the avocado in half lengthwise, and remove the pit and the peel. Place the avocado halves on your cutting board with the rounded side up.

2. Rub both halves with sushi vinegar.

3. Now, using a sharp (preferably Japanese) knife, cut thin slices (of around 4mm/⅛in) down the length of the avocado; try not to push. Turn the cutting board a quarter, and this time cut thin slices down the width of the avocado. You now have a pixelated avocado. Do you find this too difficult? Then practice first by cutting slices that are somewhat wider!

4. Carefully turn the avocados over, and use a spatula to transfer them to the toast. Season with pepper and salt.

YOU WILL NEED
cutting board
sharp knife
1 avocado
sushi vinegar
flat (metal) spatula
pepper and salt, to taste

OPTIONAL
toast

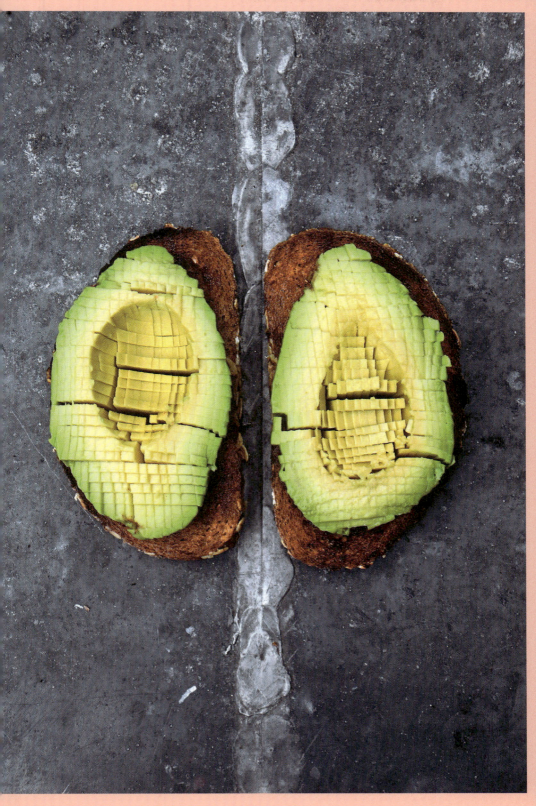

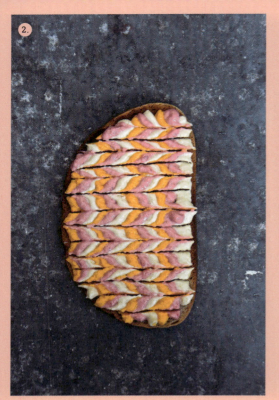

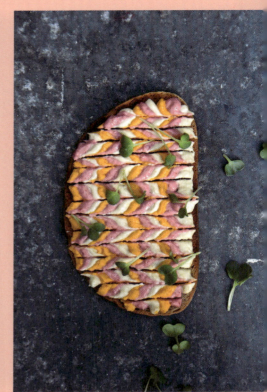

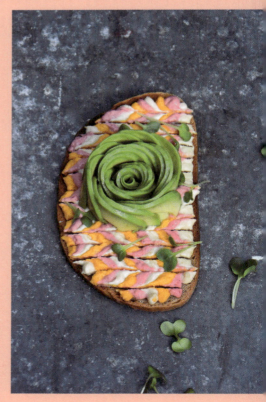

HOW TO...
MAKE A DESIGN
USING HUMMUS

1. Fill different piping bags with the various kinds of hummus. Pipe long, thin lines over the length of the toast.

2. Pull the skewer through the lines of hummus over the width of the toast. Do this every 2cm/¾in.

3. Repeat, but now pull the skewer through the lines of hummus in the opposite direction. Do this exactly in the middle of the ones you did first.

4. Garnish the toast with cress and make an avocado rose (see page 136) to place on top of the toast.

— SPREADS —
YOU CAN ALSO USE OTHER KINDS OF SAUCES OR SPREADS INSTEAD OF HUMMUS

YOU WILL NEED

2 or 3 different varieties/ colours of hummus, home-made or your favourite shop-bought kind

piping bags

toast

1 (wooden) skewer

cress

½ an avocado

TOPPINGS

edible fresh and/or dried flowers and chilli flakes (not pictured)

CREDITS

Note to readers: The tablespoons used in this book measure 15 ml, the teaspoons 5 ml. Spoons are always levelled, unless stated otherwise. Ovens work differently, always use the given temperature as a reliable indication, but adjust the cooking time and/or temperature if necessary.

| PAVILION |

First published in the United Kingdom in 2020 by
Pavilion
43 Great Ormond Street
London
WC1N 3HZ

KOS M•S MENDO

First published by Kosmos Uitgevers in the Netherlands (2018)
www.kosmosuitgevers.nl
www.mendo.nl

© 2018 The Avocado Show/MENDO.nl/Fooddeco/Kosmos Publishers, Utrecht/Antwerp
Text: The Avocado Show, Fooddeco
Recipes: Fooddeco. Inspired by The Avocado Show: page 24, 28, 50, 52, 86, 88, 110, 122, 124
Translation: Colleen Higgins, Paola Westbeek (pages 4-11)
Production assistant (Dutch Counter): Annette Doyer
Copy editor: Dieuwke de Boer
Photography & food styling: Fooddeco
Additional photography: Jet van Gaal (page 17),
Rico Franse (page 6, 7, 11), Marty Marn (page 9, top),
Kubilay Altintas (page 10, bottom), Jose da Silva (page 5, bottom),
8, 10, top, 62-63, 100-101), Ron Simpson (page 9, bottom)
Illustrations: Eddie Stok, MENDO.nl
Design: MENDO.nl

ISBN 978-1-91166-313-3

A CIP catalogue record for this book is available from the British Library.

10 9 8 7 6 5 4 3

Printed and bound by BALTO print, Lithuania

www.pavilionbooks.com